What You Need to Know about Alzheimer's Disease

Recent Titles in
Inside Diseases and Disorders

What You Need to Know about Autism
Christopher M. Cumo

What You Need to Know about ADHD
Victor B. Stolberg

What You Need to Know about ALS
Harry LeVine III

What You Need to Know about Eating Disorders
Jessica Bartley and Melissa Streno

What You Need to Know about Diabetes
Tish Davidson

What You Need to Know about the Flu
R. K. Devlin

What You Need to Know about Sleep Disorders
John T. Peachey and Diane C. Zelman

What You Need to Know about Schizophrenia
Romeo Vitelli

What You Need to Know about Asthma
Evelyn B. Kelly

What You Need to Know about Headaches
Claudio Butticè

What You Need to Know about Alzheimer's Disease

Matthew Domico and Valerie Hill

Inside Diseases and Disorders

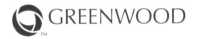

GREENWOOD

An Imprint of ABC-CLIO, LLC
Santa Barbara, California • Denver, Colorado

This book discusses treatments (including types of medication and mental health therapies), diagnostic tests for various symptoms and mental health disorders, and organizations. The authors have made every effort to present accurate and up-to-date information. However, the information in this book is not intended to recommend or endorse particular treatments or organizations, or substitute for the care or medical advice of a qualified health professional, or be used to alter any medical therapy without a medical doctor's advice. Specific situations may require specific therapeutic approaches not included in this book. For those reasons, we recommend that readers follow the advice of qualified health care professionals directly involved in their care. Readers who suspect they may have specific medical problems should consult a physician about any suggestions made in this book.

Library of Congress Cataloging-in-Publication Data

Names: Domico, Matthew, author. | Hill, Valerie, 1975- author.
Title: What you need to know about Alzheimer's disease / Matthew Domico and
   Valerie Hill.
Description: Santa Barbara, California : Greenwood, ABC-CLIO, [2022] |
   Series: Inside diseases and disorders | Includes bibliographical
   references and index.
Identifiers: LCCN 2021054204 (print) | LCCN 2021054205 (ebook) | ISBN
   9781440870316 (hardcover) | ISBN 9781440870323 (ebook)
Subjects: LCSH: Alzheimer's disease. | Families.
Classification: LCC RC523 .D66 2022 (print) | LCC RC523 (ebook) | DDC
   616.8/311—dc23/eng/20211121
LC record available at https://lccn.loc.gov/2021054204
LC ebook record available at https://lccn.loc.gov/2021054205

ISBN: 978-1-4408-7031-6 (print)
       978-1-4408-7032-3 (ebook)

26 25 24 23 22   1 2 3 4 5

This book is also available as an eBook.

Greenwood
An Imprint of ABC-CLIO, LLC

ABC-CLIO, LLC
147 Castilian Drive
Santa Barbara, California 93117
www.abc-clio.com

This book is printed on acid-free paper (∞)

Manufactured in the United States of America

To the first survivor of Alzheimer's.

Contents

Series Foreword ix

Acknowledgments xi

Introduction xiii

Essential Questions xv

CHAPTER 1
What Is Alzheimer's Disease? *1*

CHAPTER 2
The History of Alzheimer's Disease *11*

CHAPTER 3
Causes and Risk Factors *21*

CHAPTER 4
Signs and Symptoms *35*

CHAPTER 5
Diagnosis, Treatment, and Management *45*

CHAPTER 6
Long-Term Prognosis and Potential Complications *63*

CHAPTER 7
Effects on Family and Friends *77*

CHAPTER 8
Prevention *91*

CHAPTER 9
Issues and Controversies *107*

CHAPTER 10
Current Research and Future Directions *115*

Case Illustrations 135

Glossary 147

Directory of Resources 163

Bibliography 177

Index 195

Series Foreword

Disease is as old as humanity itself, and it has been the leading cause of death and disability throughout history. From the Black Death in the Middle Ages to smallpox outbreaks among Native Americans to the modern-day epidemics of diabetes and heart disease, humans have lived with—and died from—all manner of ailments, whether caused by infectious agents, environmental and lifestyle factors, or genetic abnormalities. The field of medicine has been driven forward by our desire to combat and prevent disease and to improve the lives of those living with debilitating disorders. And while we have made great strides forward, particularly in the last 100 years, it is doubtful that mankind will ever be completely free of the burden of disease.

Greenwood's Inside Diseases and Disorders series examines some of the key diseases and disorders, both physical and psychological, affecting the world today. Some (such as diabetes, cardiovascular disease, and ADHD) have been selected because of their prominence within modern America. Others (such as Ebola, celiac disease, and autism) have been chosen because they are often discussed in the media and, in some cases, are controversial or the subject of scientific or cultural debate.

Because this series covers so many different diseases and disorders, we have striven to create uniformity across all books. To maximize clarity and consistency, each book in the series follows the same format. Each begins with a collection of 10 frequently asked questions about the disease or disorder, followed by clear, concise answers. Chapter 1 provides a general introduction to the disease or disorder, including statistical information such as prevalence rates and demographic trends. The history of the disease or disorder, including how our understanding of it has evolved over time, is addressed in chapter 2. Chapter 3 examines causes and risk factors, whether genetic, microbial, or environmental, while chapter 4 discusses signs and symptoms. Chapter 5 covers the issues of diagnosis (and misdiagnosis), treatment, and management (whether with drugs, medical procedures, or lifestyle changes). How such treatment, or the lack thereof, affects a patient's long-term prognosis, as well as the risk of complications, are the subject of chapter 6. Chapter 7 explores the disease or disorder's effects on the friends and family of a patient—a dimension often overlooked in discussions of physical and psychological ailments. Chapter 8 discusses prevention strategies, while chapter 9 explores key issues or controversies, whether medical or sociocultural. Finally, chapter 10 profiles cutting-edge research and speculates on how things might change in the next few decades.

Each volume also features five fictional case studies to illustrate different aspects of the book's subject matter, highlighting key concepts and themes that have been explored throughout the text. The reader will also find a glossary of terms and a collection of print and electronic resources for additional information and further study.

As a final caveat, please be aware that the information presented in these books is no substitute for consultation with a licensed health care professional. These books do not claim to provide medical advice or guidance.

Acknowledgments

I am tremendously fortunate to have the support of so many wonderful people who provided great patience, kind understanding, and genuine interest as I worked to complete this project. I am especially grateful to my wife for helping me find time to write, for encouraging me throughout the process, and for showing me a lifetime of kindness. Thank you for every countless act of love. I am also grateful to my parents for helping me discover the path that would one day lead me to write the words printed on this page. Heartfelt thanks for everything. I would also like to express deep gratitude to my admirable colleague, Valerie Hill, for inviting me to coauthor this book. Valerie, thank you for the uplifting conversations, helpful guidance, and great camaraderie. I look forward to collaborating with you again.

—MD

This book would not have been possible without the love and support of my family and friends. I would especially like to thank my husband for his constant words of encouragement, my mother for always making sure I had uninterrupted time to write, and my "bestest" friend for always being there to lend an ear when I need it most. To my daughter, seeing your smiling face and spending time with you are by far the best part of each day. To my skillful coauthor, Matthew Domico, thank you for agreeing to take on this book with me. We were able to overcome some significant challenges and have a few laughs along the way.

—VH

Our editor, Maxine Taylor, also deserves a special thanks for being remarkably patient and helpful throughout this process. It was our pleasure to contribute to this book series.

—MD & VH

Introduction

Human development encompasses all of the changes that occur across the life span due to nature—our biological processes—and nurture—our environmental influences and life experiences. When teaching about development, we often ask students, *What is the most important developmental period: childhood, adolescence, or adulthood?* The answer given most often is "childhood." The truth is that no age period is more important than any other; each one is associated with specific milestones and unique challenges. Adulthood is comprised of various typical physical, social, and cognitive changes that naturally occur as we age; however, Alzheimer's disease is *not* one of them. But if Alzheimer's is not a typical part of normal aging, why is it ranked the sixth-leading cause of death in the United States? Alzheimer's does not only impact individuals in the United States. Instead, it is a global health epidemic that affects people all over the world. As individuals age, they or their loved ones may worry that any decline in memory or thinking ability may be due to Alzheimer's disease. This book aims to provide information about the nature of Alzheimer's, the history of the disease, its causes and risk factors, warning signs and symptoms, and how the disease is diagnosed and treated.

Alzheimer's disease is an important topic since it is currently the only major cause of death that cannot be cured, slowed down, or successfully prevented. Consequently, the mortality rate of Alzheimer's has climbed by over 145% in the United States in the last two decades. This is especially alarming when compared to changes in the mortality rates of other causes of death, such as stroke, heart disease, and HIV, which have all dropped over the last two decades. This progressive brain disease not only affects individuals living with the condition but also their loved ones. As you might expect, caring for a friend or family member living with Alzheimer's disease can be a long, demanding, and emotionally draining process. Even if we are fortunate enough to avoid the disease within our own social circles, the expected surge of Alzheimer's disease cases over the next several decades will create a global imperative that will profoundly impact our nation's health-care system, its economy, and our sociocultural understanding of the aging process. In one way or another, most people's lives will eventually be touched by the devastating consequences of Alzheimer's. We are hopeful that a more widespread understanding of the disease will pave the way for continued discussions, additional research, and new initiatives that will one day soon put an end to the terminal, incurable nature of the disease.

Essential Questions

1. WHAT IS ALZHEIMER'S DISEASE?

Alzheimer's disease is a neurodegenerative disease that causes cognitive and behavioral problems. Memory loss, for example, typically begins slowly but progresses over time, gradually becoming serious enough to disrupt everyday tasks and bodily functions. Alzheimer's disease is ultimately fatal. Refer to chapter 1 for a more complete overview of the disease.

2. WHAT IS THE DIFFERENCE BETWEEN DEMENTIA AND ALZHEIMER'S?

Dementia is a term that refers to a group of conditions characterized by a global decline in mental and physical abilities. In other words, dementia is a set of symptoms linked to a loss of memory or other cognitive abilities significant enough to impair a person's ability to carry out daily tasks. Alzheimer's disease is the most severe, devastating, and common form of dementia. Chapter 1 defines dementia, Alzheimer's disease, and Alzheimer's dementia in greater detail and discusses the differences between them.

3. WHAT ARE THE RISK FACTORS FOR ALZHEIMER'S?

The greatest known risk factor is increasing age; however, it is important to remember that Alzheimer's is not a typical part of aging. Other risk factors include family history, apolipoprotein E (APOE) ε4 gene, smoking, obesity, high blood pressure, high cholesterol, sedentary lifestyle, education level, and stress. Chapter 3 discusses each of these risk factors.

4. HOW DO I KNOW IF MY LOVED ONE HAS ALZHEIMER'S?

Symptoms of the disease (e.g., memory loss, decline in the ability to perform routine tasks, impairment of judgment) develop slowly and gradually. Therefore, the disease process can begin years before an individual notices any changes. In addition, there is no single test to determine whether someone has Alzheimer's. Instead, doctors use a multifaceted approach that often includes a complete medical history (including family history of the disease), physical examination, laboratory and cognitive tests, brain-imaging tools, as well discussing any changes in thinking and/or everyday behaviors. Refer to chapter 4 for more information about the signs and symptoms of the disease and chapter 5 for how the disease is diagnosed.

5. WHEN CAN SOMEONE DEVELOP ALZHEIMER'S?

The majority of people with Alzheimer's are age 65 or older; this is called late-onset Alzheimer's. Only up to 5% of individuals with Alzheimer's have early-onset Alzheimer's. This type happens to people who are younger than age 65. Often, they are in their 40s or 50s when they are diagnosed with the disease. Most people who have early-onset Alzheimer's have familial Alzheimer's disease (FAD). Doctors know that this form of the disease is linked to genes; at least two generations of their family have had the disease. For more information, see chapter 1 regarding the prevalence rate of the disease and chapter 3 for the timing of early versus late onset.

6. WHAT ARE THE CAUSES OF ALZHEIMER'S?

There are many factors that contribute to someone developing Alzheimer's. Specific genetic mutations are typically linked to the development of Alzheimer's disease in people who experience it early in life. A mixture of genetic, lifestyle, and environmental factors are believed to contribute to the risk of developing Alzheimer's disease later in life. Refer to chapter 3 for more detailed information regarding the potential causes of Alzheimer's.

7. HOW IS ALZHEIMER'S TREATED?

Alzheimer's disease is complex, and no single drug or intervention is likely to be effective in treating it. Current treatments are aimed at assisting patients in maintaining mental function, managing behavioral symptoms, and slowing the progression of disease symptoms. Several prescription drugs are currently approved by the Food and Drug Administration (FDA) to treat people who have been diagnosed with Alzheimer's disease: Razadyne®, Exelon®, and Aricept® among others. Individuals with Alzheimer's disease will be able to live with comfort, dignity, and freedom for a longer period of time if their symptoms are treated. Most drugs are most effective when used by people who are in the early or middle stages of the disease. For example, drugs may temporarily slow down symptoms such as memory loss. It is important to note, however, that none of these drugs will stop the disease itself. Refer to chapters 2 and 5 for a more detailed explanation of these as well as other approaches used to treat the disease.

8. IS THERE A CURE FOR ALZHEIMER'S?

Alzheimer's disease currently has no cure, although there are treatments for the symptoms, and research is ongoing to find new ways to treat the disease, postpone its progression, and prevent it from developing. Refer to chapter 5 for management of the disease and chapter 8 regarding prevention.

9. WHAT IS THE DURATION OF THE DISEASE?

An individual with Alzheimer's disease lives on average 4 to 8 years after diagnosis but can survive for up to 20 years depending on other factors. Refer to chapter 6 for information regarding prognosis and course of the disease.

10. HOW CAN I CARE FOR A LOVED ONE SUFFERING FROM ALZHEIMER'S?

Caring for loved ones who are living with Alzheimer's or some other type of dementia can be a long, stressful, and emotional journey. The type of care needed for your loved ones depends on which stage of the disease they are in (i.e., mild, moderate, or severe). The more you learn about the disease and its progression over time, the better prepared you will be. Overall, it is helpful to develop a personal support plan, adapt to changes in communication (e.g., keep communication short and simple, speak slowly, use close-ended questions, and repeat information when necessary), and develop daily routines. Chapter 7 discusses in greater detail the role caregivers play in taking care of a loved one who is living with the disease.

1

What Is Alzheimer's Disease?

Every 65 seconds, someone in the United States develops Alzheimer's disease, a debilitating neurological disorder that progressively deteriorates memory, cognitive functioning, and behavior. According to 2021 statistics provided by the Centers for Disease Control and Prevention (CDC), Alzheimer's disease is ranked as the sixth-leading cause of death in the United States, and it surpasses the number of yearly deaths caused by diabetes, kidney disease, influenza, and suicide. In fact, Alzheimer's disease is the only one of the top 10 leading causes of death that cannot be cured, slowed down, or reliably prevented. Health scientists have demonstrated that Alzheimer's disease is a significant global health epidemic, and rising statistics foreshadow a challenging future. Over the past two decades, the mortality rate of Alzheimer's disease in the United States *increased* by 145.2%—a finding that is especially concerning when viewed alongside the mortality rate trajectories of other leading causes of death (such as stroke, HIV, and heart disease), which have *decreased* over the last 20 years. Consistent with the rising death rate, the number of people currently living with Alzheimer's disease is expected to skyrocket over the next several years. In 2021, an estimated 6.2 million Americans have Alzheimer's disease, but by 2025, that number is projected to grow by 16% to 7.2 million. By 2060, the total number of people with Alzheimer's disease is expected to reach a staggering 13.8 million.

THE DIFFERENCE BETWEEN DEMENTIA, ALZHEIMER'S DISEASE, AND ALZHEIMER'S DEMENTIA

The word *dementia* is derived from the Latin word *demens*, meaning "without mind." Dementia is not a specific disease; it is a general term that is used to categorize several types of brain diseases in which a person experiences a gradual decline in one or more cognitive abilities. Memory loss is the most common deficit, but individuals with dementia can also experience progressive losses in thinking, orientation, calculation, learning capacity, language, and judgment. Importantly, dementia does not produce a clouding of consciousness—in other words, it does not alter the person's level of wakefulness or their awareness of their surroundings. The cognitive deficits that are observed in dementia are often accompanied (or preceded) by emotional and behavioral impairments, which can include a lack of motivation, difficulty controlling one's emotions, or inappropriate behavior around others. Although some of these difficulties can be expected as normal outcomes of advanced aging, dementia symptoms are more pervasive and severe. A diagnosis of dementia is only made when individuals' cognitive decline becomes so incapacitating that they are no longer able to perform complex daily living skills by themselves, such as paying bills, managing medications, or acquiring/cooking meals.

Alzheimer's disease is the most severe, devastating, and common form of dementia, accounting for 60% to 80% of all dementia cases. Alzheimer's disease features the same observable symptoms as all forms of dementia; however, the term *Alzheimer's disease* is only used when cognitive decline is believed to originate from the destruction of cells found in parts of the brain that are important for memory and other cognitive functions. Cellular destruction in Alzheimer's disease occurs because of the presence of two hallmark forms of pathophysiology that distinguish Alzheimer's disease from other dementias. The first is amyloid plaques, clusters of fragmented proteins that form between brain cells. These sticky, abnormal clumps block communication between the brain's nerve cells, and their presence triggers the immune system to attack and destroy nerve cells that have been enveloped by the plaques. A second indicator of Alzheimer's disease, neurofibrillary tangles, are twisted strands of protein found within nerve cells. They prevent nutrients from moving through cells, leading the cells to collapse and disintegrate. Together, these two destructive processes spread throughout the brain in a predictable pattern, causing cell death and widespread brain deterioration. By the late stages of disease, the brain will lose a significant amount of its total volume, and nearly all of its functions will be severely impaired.

A definitive diagnosis of Alzheimer's disease can only be made posthumously, after medical professionals confirm the presence of the characteristic plaques and tangles within the diseased tissues of an autopsied brain. The term *Alzheimer's dementia* is used in situations where Alzheimer's disease is the most likely cause of a patient's symptoms but biological detection methods have not been used to confirm the presence of Alzheimer's disease pathophysiology. There is good reason for the ubiquity of this careful labeling: several autopsy studies have confirmed that as many as 30% of individuals who fit the diagnostic criteria for the disease, based on clinical symptoms, did not actually have Alzheimer's-related brain changes. Fortunately, new methods are currently being developed to identify the biological presence of plaques and tangles through noninvasive means, allowing for earlier and more conclusive diagnoses (see chapter 10).

Several types of dementia exist in addition to Alzheimer's disease. Vascular dementia, which occurs after a stroke, is the second most common dementia type. Other common causes of dementia include cerebrovascular disease, Lewy body disease, and Parkinson's disease (see chapter 5). However, it is important to note there are several other conditions that can cause symptoms that resemble dementia, such as thyroid problems, certain vitamin deficiencies, depression, untreated sleep apnea, and excessive alcohol consumption. In contrast to Alzheimer's disease, these conditions can often be reversed with successful treatment. Besides dementia, there are other brain conditions such as traumatic brain injury (TBI), mild cognitive impairment (MCI), and chronic traumatic encephalopathy (CTE) that can cause problems with memory, thinking, and behavior. For instance, TBI results from a sudden impact to the head that causes nondegenerative injury to the brain, which can temporarily or permanently impair a person's cognitive and psychosocial functions. Individuals who suffer from this condition experience a reduced or altered state of consciousness that is not observed in Alzheimer's disease. MCI produces a slight but perceivable decline in memory and thinking skills but not to the extent that independent living and the ability to perform daily life skills are compromised. In contrast to Alzheimer's disease, many people with MCI do not experience a continued progression of cognitive decline, and a substantial number of MCI patients across several studies have been shown to make a full recovery. Even so, a person who suffers from MCI is more likely to ultimately develop Alzheimer's disease or another form of dementia. CTE is a condition that may develop after repeated injuries to the head and is most common in athletes and military veterans. It is linked to several symptoms similar to Alzheimer's disease, such as confusion, memory problems, cognitive difficulties, and emotional changes. Unlike Alzheimer's disease, CTE develops much earlier in the life span, and it directly results from physical injury; no one has ever been diagnosed with CTE without having a history of head trauma.

PREVALENCE AND INCIDENCE

Alzheimer's disease affects the lives of millions of people across the world, and unfortunately, it is widely expected that the number and proportion of people living with the disease will continue to grow at an alarming rate, especially as the population of Americans age 65 and older increases from 58 million in 2021 to a projected 98 million in 2060. Alzheimer's disease presents a significant risk to many Americans, and epidemiological research elucidates the pervasiveness of the disease and offers some indications of one's risk of developing the disease at different points throughout middle and late adulthood. Health scientists commonly use two different measures of disease frequency to describe how often a disease occurs within a population. *Prevalence rate* represents the proportion of existing cases of disease in a population at a given time. It is often used to predict the burden that a disease has on particular nation or geographic region in terms of economic strain, quality of life, and other factors. *Incidence rate* measures the number of new cases of disease within a specific time period. It provides an estimate of how quickly a disease occurs within a population, and it is often used to determine one's risk of developing a disease.

Some researchers have used prevalence statistics to predict the total number of people in the United States who have Alzheimer's disease. Of the estimated 6.2 million Americans living with Alzheimer's disease in 2021, 28% are between the ages of 65 and 75, 36% are between the ages of 75 and 84, and the remaining 36% are over age 85. These findings, presented in the *Journal of the Alzheimer's Association*, are based on the outcome of a longitudinal research study that categorized people as having Alzheimer's disease if they demonstrated clinical symptoms of the disease. Other researchers have estimated the proportion of diseased individuals within the entire U.S. population. Data from the Aging, Demographics, and Memory Study (ADAMS), which used a representative sample of adults from across the United States, concluded that 11.3% of all Americans over the age of 65 are living with Alzheimer's disease in 2021. In other words, one out of every nine people over the age of 65 is believed to develop, and eventually die from, the disease. Although these numbers are already large enough to raise concern, researchers believe that the number of people who actually have Alzheimer's disease is significantly higher than what prevalence estimates currently indicate. That's because Alzheimer's disease prevalence statistics do not include patients who experience MCI, a condition that sometimes progresses into Alzheimer's disease. In the near future, new biomarker assessment technologies will likely allow researchers to identify, with near certainty, which MCI patients actually have early-stage Alzheimer's disease and which ones do not.

Because there are over 5 million people over the age of 65 who have MCI, and about half of them are expected to develop full-blown Alzheimer's disease, it is therefore likely that the true number of Americans who are currently living with some level of Alzheimer's disease is well over 6.2 million.

Regarding the incidence of Alzheimer's disease, researchers have estimated that approximately 910,000 people over the age of 65 developed the progressive neurological disorder in 2011. This estimate was first reported by a group of researchers in 2019, who made incidence predictions by utilizing 2010 U.S. Census data in addition to findings from the large-scale Chicago Health and Aging Project (CHAP) study. CHAP is a widely cited, 19-year longitudinal investigation that collected neurocognitive data from 10,801 older adults living on the South Side of Chicago between 1993 and 2012. The 2019 researchers who utilized CHAP data to make estimates about the 2011 incidence have suggested that the number of annual Alzheimer's disease cases would likely be even higher in 2020 if CHAP estimates were available for that year. CHAP incidence rates further indicate that new cases of Alzheimer's disease increase significantly as people age. For example, in 2011, the average annual incidence for people between 65 and 74 years old was predicted to be 3 afflicted people out of every 1,000 individuals. But as people aged to between 75 and 84 years of age, the incidence rate increased *tenfold* to 32 cases out of every 1,000. Finally, among the nation's "oldest old," the projected incidence reached an alarming proportion of 76 out of 1,000. Clearly, age is a great risk factor for the development of Alzheimer's disease, but as we will see in chapter 6, Alzheimer's disease is not a typical or expected outcome of the normal aging process. In other words, old age predicts greater likelihood of developing Alzheimer's, but it does not cause the disease.

Sex Differences

More women than men are living with Alzheimer's disease in the United States. Out of the 6.2 million people who are expected to have the disease, 3.8 million are expected to be women. The reason for this disparity could be due to the fact that women, on average, tend to outlive men by about five years and old age is the greatest risk factor for developing the incurable brain disease. If more women lived into the later stages of the human life span, it could explain why a greater number of women are predicted to have Alzheimer's disease. Several research studies on U.S. populations have concluded that when men and women of the same age group are examined, both sexes show comparable incidence rates. However, a different conclusion was reached by researchers who conducted a 2018 meta-analysis that examined 298 publications between 2016 and 2017 from the United States, Europe, and Asia. Their review concluded that women suffer from greater cognitive deterioration than men, even when the two sexes are compared at the same age and the same stage of disease. In other words, the longer life span of women did not account for the increased incidence. The researchers also found evidence that when age and disease severity were held constant, women with Alzheimer's disease showed greater impairment across several cognitive domains, including semantic memory (remembering facts), episodic memory (recalling personal experiences), visual processing (the brain's ability to convert light energy to meaningful images), and verbal processing (the ability to send and receive ideas through written and oral communication). Geographic region was speculated to play a role in explaining these differences.

Various societal, cultural, and biological differences may predispose women to have a greater risk of developing dementia and suffering from its effects. Some researchers have suggested that education level may be a factor that could explain the difference. Women who were born in the first half of the twentieth century typically did not attain the same level of education as their male counterparts, and therefore, a lack of formal learning could be responsible for elevating one's risk of developing age-related cognitive decline. Research collected in the United States suggests that increases in educational attainment over time are linked to lower dementia rates. However, educational differences between men and women may not fully explain why women are more vulnerable to developing dementia. A European study found that lower levels of education predicted the development of Alzheimer's disease in women but not in men, even when researchers controlled for variables such as social class, psychological stress, and occupation. This suggests that other factors, in addition to educational attainment, need to be considered to more fully understand why woman have a greater risk of developing cognitive decline. Other research has examined the role of genetic and biological factors that could more fully explain women's heightened susceptibility to developing Alzheimer's pathology. The APOE ε4 genotype, the most reliable genetic risk indicator of Alzheimer's disease, is more strongly associated with greater brain atrophy and cognitive impairment among women than among men who share the same gene variant. Likewise, women typically show more accelerated cognitive decline even when they have the similar levels of the telltale biological signs of Alzheimer's disease: amyloid plaques and hyperphosphorylated tau (a pathological form of a protein that builds inside of nerve cells in the brain and causes neurofibrillary tangles). That these characteristic features of Alzheimer's disease seem to take a more detrimental toll on women than on men is possibly due to the sex hormone estrogen, which has been shown to activate the APOE ε4 gene variant. Researchers are still exploring other mechanisms that could contribute to the sex differences in dementia rates.

Racial/Ethnic Differences

Alzheimer's disease affects the lives of more whites than any other racial group in the United States, simply because whites are the largest racial group in the country. However, when future demographic projections and proportional data about dementia rates in minority groups are examined, a different and more troubling picture is brought into focus. According to U.S. Census estimates for 2020, Blacks and Hispanic Americans only made up a combined total of 19% of the nation's elderly (65 years and older) population. But by 2060, these two minority groups will make up a combined total of 35% of the elderly demographic in the United States. This projection, coupled with the widely held expectation that Alzheimer's rates will dramatically increase over the next several decades, calls attention to an interesting line of research that examines the link between race/ethnicity and the risk of developing Alzheimer's disease. Multiple investigations, dating from 1997 to 2020, have revealed that Alzheimer's disease disproportionately affects Black and Hispanic Americans. According to a 2020 report from the American Alzheimer's Association, African Americans are about twice as likely to have Alzheimer's disease, and Hispanics are about 1.5 times more likely to develop the condition. Interestingly, genetic factors are not believed to account for the difference. Instead, comorbid medical conditions, socioeconomic factors, and other health conditions seem to better explain the disparity. For example, high blood pressure and diabetes, which are known risk factors for Alzheimer's disease, are more widely experienced by Black and Hispanic Americans. These minority groups are also at higher risk for poverty, violence, discrimination, and lower educational attainment, factors that are believed to play a significant role in the development of dementia across the life span. A few research studies have found that Black Americans who grow up experiencing segregation in schools or who report detrimental living conditions early in life tend to have diminished cognitive health as adults. When researchers examined racial/ethnic differences after controlling for the influence of comorbid health conditions and socioeconomic factors, the differences in dementia rates between white and minority populations were no longer present. These findings suggest that improved health-care management within Black and Hispanic American communities may help decrease the disproportional impact of dementia on these racial/ethnic groups.

MYTHS ABOUT THE DISEASE

There are a variety of myths associated with aging and specifically Alzheimer's. According to the Alzheimer's Association, some of the most commons myths people believe to be true are (1) memory loss is a natural part of aging, (2) Alzheimer's disease is not fatal, (3) only older people can get Alzheimer's, (4) flu shots increase the risk of Alzheimer's disease, and (5) there are treatments available to stop the progression of Alzheimer's disease.

Memory loss is not a typical part of aging. As people age, it is not out of the ordinary to experience occasional memory problems such as forgetting the name of someone they recently met. However, individuals with Alzheimer's have more than occasional memory loss. Since Alzheimer's disease causes brain cells to malfunction and eventually die, these individuals may forget the name of a loved one or how to get home from a grocery store they have frequented for many years. In addition, Alzheimer's disease is fatal: no one has ever survived Alzheimer's. It slowly takes away a person's identity, ability to communicate with others, ability to think and remember, and ability to perform everyday activities that most adults take for granted, such as eating, getting dressed, or going to the bathroom. It is also a myth that only elderly people can get Alzheimer's. Alzheimer's can devastate the lives of people in their 30s, 40s, and 50s, although it is uncommon. When this happens, it is called early-onset Alzheimer's disease. It is estimated that approximately 200,000 people younger than age 65 have early-onset Alzheimer's, which is far less than the estimated 6.2 million people in the United States who are believed to experience the disease at the age of 65 and over. Early- versus late-onset Alzheimer's disease will be discussed further in chapter 3. It is also a myth that flu shots increase the risk of Alzheimer's disease. A theory linking flu shots to an increased risk of Alzheimer's disease, proposed by a U.S. doctor whose license was later suspended by the South Carolina Board of Medical Examiners, is believed to be the main reason for the existence of this myth. Actually, research shows the opposite: there are several studies that link flu shots and other vaccinations to a reduced risk of Alzheimer's disease. For example, in 2001, the *Canadian Medical Association Journal* (*CMAJ*) published an article that found adults who were vaccinated against diphtheria, tetanus, poliomyelitis, and influenza had a lower risk of developing Alzheimer's disease than those who had not received those vaccinations. This shows that past exposure to vaccines may protect against subsequent development of Alzheimer's disease. Similarly, in 2004, a report in the *Journal of the American Medical Association* (*JAMA*) found that annual flu shots for older adults were linked to a reduced risk of death from all causes. The final myth is that there are treatments to stop the progression of the disease. At this point in time, there is no treatment to cure, delay, or stop the progression of Alzheimer's disease. Drugs approved by the Food and Drug Administration (FDA) temporarily slow the worsening of symptoms for about 6 to 12 months, on average, for about half of the individuals who take them, but none of them cures, delays, or stops the disease currently. The treatment and management of Alzheimer's disease will be described in greater detail in chapter 5.

2

The History of Alzheimer's Disease

As discussed in chapter 1, Alzheimer's disease is a degenerative brain disease that causes a gradual and irreversible loss of brain functions such as memory, language skills, perception, loss of the ability to care for oneself, and eventually the loss of basic bodily functions such as walking and swallowing. In this chapter, we will take a look at the history of the disease, including who discovered the disease, when the disease was discovered, and what progress has been made since its discovery.

DISCOVERY OF THE DISEASE

Alzheimer's disease is named after the individual who is credited for having discovered the disease: Alois Alzheimer, a German psychiatrist. An article titled "Alzheimer and His Disease" in the journal *Neurological Sciences* gives an overview of his life and work. Alois was born into a Catholic family on June 14, 1864, in the small town of Marktbreit close to Würzburg on the River Main in Germany. His father's first wife had died two years before Alois was born, leaving one son. The father, Edward, then married his first child's aunt, Therese Busch. Alois was the firstborn of Edward and Therese Alzheimer. Alois went to elementary school in Marktbreit and to secondary school in Aschaffenburg. Following secondary study in Aschaffenburg, he studied medicine in Berlin, Tübingen, and

Würzburg. At the time, he was not interested in psychiatry; rather, he studied anatomy and learned to work with microscopes. In 1887, he defended his doctoral dissertation on the ceruminous glands of the ear.

After he earned his degree in medicine, according to the article, "The Discovery of Alzheimer's Disease," in *Dialogues of Clinical Neuroscience*, he went to work for a wealthy German family and traveled with them to take care of one of their "mentally ill" relatives. That was the practice at that time of some very wealthy families in Germany: to have a young medical doctor travel with the "patient." Alzheimer traveled for approximately five months with such a family and took care of one of their female relatives. It was through that experience that Alzheimer gained interest in clinical psychiatry.

Upon returning in fall of 1888, Alzheimer began his medical career as a resident at the Municipal Asylum for the Mentally Ill and Epileptics in Frankfurt, Germany. He had a variety of research interests, including epilepsy, the degenerative and vascular origins of dementia, forensic psychiatry, and contraception. During his time at the hospital, Alzheimer met Franz Nissl who, a few years earlier, developed a new staining technique, which is still used today, for examining parts of the nervous system under a microscope. Together, they began to conduct research on the pathology of the nervous system, in particular, the anatomy of the cerebral cortex. Alzheimer's focus was on linking mental illness with results he obtained from postmortem tests on the brain.

In 1894, Alois married a wealthy widow named Cecilie Geisenheimer. The couple had three children: Gertrud, Hans, and Maria. In 1901, shortly after the birth of their third child, Cecilie passed away. With three young children to take care of, Alois asked his younger sister, who was not married, to come live with him to help raise his children and take care of the household. To help cope with his grief over the loss of his wife, Alois immersed himself in his work. He focused on the treatment of patients with mental illness and conducted research at the Community Hospital for Mental and Epileptic Patients, in Frankfurt, Germany. Even though his income from his position at the hospital was not much, because of the wealth he acquired while married to Cecilie, he could devote himself to his work without worrying about money. Dr. Alzheimer was a hardworking, young psychiatrist who was committed to understanding the relationship between diseases of the brain and mental illness. Alzheimer saw all newly admitted patients and extensively documented his findings. On November 25, 1901, a new patient by the name of Auguste Deter was admitted to the Frankfurt hospital.

According to the article, "History of Alzheimer's Disease," in the journal *Dementia and Neurocognitive Disorders*, Auguste was born on May 16, 1850, in Kassel, Germany, into a working-class family. She was relatively well educated for being from a poor family. At the age of 14, she started working as a seamstress assistant. Auguste met Karl Deter and married him at the age of 23. They moved to Frankfurt, where Karl worked for a railway company. They had a daughter and lived a relatively ordinary life until early 1901. Auguste was only 50 years old when her husband noticed changes in her behavior. She intentionally hid things around the house and had trouble sleeping, writing, and cooking meals. Besides these behaviors, Karl also noticed her increasing memory problems. Auguste struggled to remember where she was and how to have a conversation. She soon became fearful, paranoid, and aggressive, making it necessary for her husband to admit her to the psychiatric hospital. On November 26, 1901, at the age of 51, Auguste was examined by Alzheimer.

Alzheimer began by assessing Auguste's demeanor, asking her very simple questions, and systematically writing down her answers. The article, "Auguste D and Alzheimer's Disease," in *The Lancet*, gives a detailed account of Alzheimer's handwritten notes regarding Auguste Deter. For example, on November 26, 1901, Alzheimer noted that Auguste was sitting in the bed with a helpless expression on her face. He asked, "'What is your name?' Auguste answered, 'Auguste.' 'Last name?' 'Auguste.' 'What is your husband's name?' 'Auguste, I think.' 'Your husband?' 'Ah, my husband.'" Alzheimer noted that Auguste looked as if she did not understand the questions he was asking her. He went on to ask, "'Are you married?' Auguste answered, 'To Auguste.' 'Mrs. D?' 'Yes, yes, Auguste D.' 'How long have you been here?' 'Three weeks.'" Then Alzheimer showed Auguste a variety of objects to see if she knew what they were: pencil, purse, key, diary, and cigar. She was able to identify all of the objects but the pencil; she called it a pen. Alzheimer went on to write that at lunch, Auguste was eating pork with a side of cauliflower and, when asked what she was eating, she replied, "Spinach." "When she was chewing meat and was asked what she was doing, she answered, 'potatoes' and then 'horseradish.'" Alzheimer also noted that when objects were shown to Auguste, she could not recall them after a brief period of time. In addition, she had difficulty writing. When asked to write her name, she tried writing "Mrs" and then forgot the rest. He also noted that words had to be continually repeated to her. Alzheimer observed her on several days afterward and diagnosed her condition as "presenile dementia." Presenile dementia refers to dementia before the age of 65.

Alzheimer wanted to continue to assess Auguste; however, the medical expenses were too much for her husband to cover. Therefore, Alzheimer arranged for Auguste to stay at the hospital in exchange for her medical records and brain when she passed away. Her husband Karl agreed and signed the consent for Alzheimer to acquire those when Auguste died. Over the years, Auguste's condition deteriorated. She mumbled to herself, could not get out of bed without assistance, and had difficulty doing simple daily activities such as eating without help. Auguste remained an inpatient at that community hospital until her death. In the end, she lost all cognitive ability and died of pneumonia on April 8, 1906, although by then she was no longer under Dr. Alzheimer's care. He had since taken a research position at the Munich Hospital under the leadership of Dr. Emil Kraepelin. Today, Kraepelin is often recognized as the "father of scientific psychiatry." Alzheimer's former boss from Frankfurt, Dr. Emil Sioli, informed Dr. Alzheimer of Auguste Deter's death. He sent her medical records and brain material to Alzheimer, who examined her brain microscopically. Alzheimer applied a staining technique that revealed, for the first time, the presence of what are now called amyloid plaques and neurofibrillary tangles. Dr. Alzheimer wrote in the autopsy that Auguste had shrinkage in and around nerve cells in her brain. The cerebral cortex was thinned, and the region that is involved with thinking, memory, judgment, and language was severely impaired.

Dr. Kraepelin saw Alzheimer's work and encouraged him to present his findings. Therefore, on November 3, 1906, Alzheimer gave a lecture at the 37th Conference of the Southwest German Psychiatrists, in Tübingen. In his lecture, he described a patient by the name of Auguste D, a 51-year-old female who had shown gradual cognitive impairment, hallucinations, delusions, and lack of understanding regarding social situations. He noted that these abnormal symptoms were produced in the cerebral cortex. However, the presentation did not attract any attention or comments, and no questions were asked at the end of his lecture. Psychoanalytic studies presented at the meeting received more attention than Alzheimer's and were the ones to get reported in the local press. Alzheimer was disappointed he did not receive attention from renowned scholars, who most likely assumed Alzheimer was discussing a neurodegenerative disorder that was rare and only afflicted a few people during middle age.

The following year, he published his presentation under the title, "A Characteristic Serious Disease of the Cerebral Cortex." The article, "Auguste D and Alzheimer's Disease," in *The Lancet*, describes what Alzheimer wrote (without identifying Auguste): "[A] 51-year-old woman who showed as one of her first disease symptoms a strong feeling of jealousy toward her husband. Very soon she showed rapidly increasing memory impairments; she was disoriented carrying objects to and fro in her flat and hid them. Sometimes she felt that someone wanted to kill her and began to scream loudly. . . . After 4½ years of sickness she died." The article continues by explaining some of his other findings. "He reported peculiar changes in the neurofibrils: 'In the centre of an otherwise almost normal cell there stands out one or several fibrils due to their characteristic thickness and peculiar impregnability.' He also described the typical plaques:

'Numerous small military foci are found in the superior layers. They are determined by the storage of a peculiar material in the cortex.'" In his writings, Alzheimer did not name the disease after himself. Instead, Dr. Emil Kraepelin, coined the term "Alzheimer's disease" in the eighth edition (which was published in 1910) of the *Handbook of Psychiatry*. Alzheimer and others were surprised that Kraepelin had named the condition "Alzheimer's disease," but nevertheless, the name stuck. It is thought that Kraepelin had probably named the disease after Alzheimer to give his institution more prestige and to ensure the continuation of research funding for the laboratory. According to the article, "History of Alzheimer's Disease," in *Dementia and Neurocognitive Disorders*, there were two competing institutions investigating neuropathology at that time. One was in Munich under the leadership of Emil Kraepelin, and the other was in Prague under the leadership of Arnold Pick. When Alzheimer reported the pathological features of senile plaques and neurofibrillary tangles, Oskar Fisher, from the Prague institution, had already mentioned senile plaques in one of his patients.

Alois Alzheimer died five years later, on December 19, 1915, from an infection of the heart, not knowing his surname would become a household name.

AWARENESS OF THE DISEASE

As described in chapter 1, the word *dementia* is an overall term that describes a category of conditions that involve global deterioration in intellectual abilities and physical function. The term can be traced back to the time of ancient Greece and Rome, where it was considered a typical and inevitable part of aging. Geras Solutions is a company that aims to improve the lives of millions who have been directly or indirectly affected by cognitive decline or dementia by providing access to remote care with the help of digitized diagnostic and supportive solutions. It is cleverly named "Geras" after the Greek god of old age. According to definitions. net, it was once believed that the more "geras" one acquired, the more fame and courage the person was supposed to have, but despite this protection, people were still susceptible to cognitive decline. We can see dementia being referred to by other famous Greek individuals. For instance, Pythagoras, a Greek physician of the seventh century BCE, divided the life cycle into six stages: infancy (ages 0–6), adolescence (ages 7–21), adulthood (ages 22–49), middle age (ages 50–62), senescence (ages 63–79), and old age (ages 80 and above). He believed the last two life cycle stages, senescence and old age, were mostly identified by the decline of the human body and mental abilities. Similarly, Hippocrates, who lived between the third and fourth centuries BCE and who many consider to be the "father of medicine," also spoke about the deterioration of mind due to old age. He also believed that brain injury resulted in cognitive disorder. Famous Greek philosophers Plato and Aristotle, who also lived around that time, thought mental and cognitive decline were an unavoidable consequence of getting older.

Greeks were not the only ones writing about old age. Marcus Cicero, a Roman philosopher who lived in the second century BCE, was one of the first to suggest that dementia was not an inevitable consequence of aging. He pointed out that aging does not always cause the decline of mental performance. Also, Galen, an influential Roman physician, who lived in the second century CE, wrote about dementia, using the term *morosis*, including it in his list of mental diseases and indicating it may occur in old age. According to the article, "History of Alzheimer's Disease" in *Dementia and Neurocognitive Disorders*, in the modern age, dementia as a diagnosis was initially accepted as a medical term in 1797 by French physician Philippe Pinel. Back then, those living with a mental disease were confined to asylums and not treated very well. This started to change in the nineteenth century mainly due to Pinel, who advocated for a more humanitarian way of treating and caring for individuals who suffered from mental illness. Improving the conditions in which these individuals lived also provided better settings for clinical observation.

In 1894, Otto Binswanger, a Swiss scientist, and Alzheimer published a report on neurosyphilis, one of the causes of dementia. In the report, the term *presenile dementia* made its first appearance. As mentioned in the previous section, in 1901, after Alzheimer observed Auguste Deter for several days, he diagnosed her with having "presenile dementia." In 1910, psychiatrist Emil Kraepelin classified dementia into "senile dementia" and "presenile dementia" in the *Handbook of Psychiatry* (where, as stated earlier, he was the first to refer to "Alzheimer's disease"). By studying the brain of his former patient, Auguste Deter, Alzheimer reported having discovered pathological features of "presenile dementia."

After the 1910 publication mentioning Alzheimer's disease, it went relatively ignored until decades later. Why this happened is not quite clear. Along with the idea that Alzheimer's disease was thought of as relatively rare was the fact that studying clinical symptoms through anatomy was not widely practiced.

The Alzheimer's Association and a 2018 article in the *International Journal of Engineering and Creative Science* highlight the major milestones regarding the disease. The following is a timeline of advancements related to awareness, research, and treatments for Alzheimer's disease since its discovery.

1931: Max Knoll, a German electrical engineer, and Ernst Ruska, a German physicist, invent the electron microscope. This microscope replaces regular microscopes, allowing scientists to view objects closer up through greater magnification. This invention allows scientists to see the fine details of objects and study the interior structures of cells. However, the electron microscope will not become readily available in research settings until after World War II.

1968: Researchers develop the first valid cognitive measurement scale for assessing cognitive and physical decline in older adults, thus allowing researchers to measure impairment and estimate the amount of damaged brain tissue.

1974: Congress establishes the National Institute on Aging (NIA) as one of the National Institutes of Health (NIH). To this day, the NIA is the primary federal agency that supports Alzheimer's research.

1976: In an editorial published in the medical journal *Archives of Neurology*, Robert Katzman identifies Alzheimer's disease as the most common cause of dementia.

1980: The Alzheimer's Association is established. In the previous year, Jerome H. Stone, along with individuals from numerous family support groups, met with the NIA to discuss the importance of a national, independent, nonprofit organization to aid federal efforts on Alzheimer's disease. As a result, the Alzheimer's Association is formed, with Stone as the founding president. Today, the Alzheimer's Association is the leading voluntary health organization connected with Alzheimer's disease.

1983: Congress declares November 1983 the first National Alzheimer's Disease Month, indicating a greater awareness of the disease. Each year in November, the aim is to make the general public more aware of the disease and its prevalence among the U.S. population. In 1983, fewer than 2 million individuals were diagnosed with the disease. Currently, approximately 5.8 million individuals in the United States are living with the disease.

1984: Beta-amyloid is identified. Researchers George Glenner and Cai'ne Wong report identification of "a novel cerebrovascular amyloid protein," known as beta-amyloid. This is the main component of Alzheimer's senile plaques and a key contributor to nerve cell damage.

1984: The NIA begins to fund Alzheimer's Disease Centers and establishes a nationwide network for Alzheimer's research, diagnosis, and treatment.

1986: Belgian physician Jean Pierre Brion identifies the tau protein as a key component of neurofibrillary tangles, the second pathological hallmark of Alzheimer's disease and another key aspect in nerve cell degeneration.

1987: Alzheimer's first drug trial is conducted. The Alzheimer's Association assists the NIA and the Warner-Lambert Pharmaceutical Company (now Pfizer) in launching and recruiting participants for clinical trials of tacrine, the first drug specifically targeting symptoms of Alzheimer's disease. That same year, the first Alzheimer's gene is identified. The gene, located on chromosome 21, codes amyloid precursor protein (APP), the parent molecule from which beta-amyloid is formed. It is the first gene with mutations found to cause a rare, inherited form of Alzheimer's disease.

1990: Winfried Denk and James Strickler at Cornell University develop a technique called two-photon microscopy. Two-photon microscopy has permitted scientists to understand changes in a living brain during everyday processes such as learning, as well as changes that occur over the course of a disease—for example, witnessing how the branches on neurons near senile plaques associated with Alzheimer's break down over time.

1991: The NIA establishes the Alzheimer's Disease Cooperative Study (ADCS), which is a nationwide medical network to facilitate clinical research and conduct federally funded clinical trials.

1992: Presenilin 1 is identified as the second gene with mutations found to be associated with a rare, inherited form of Alzheimer's disease.

1993: Presenilin 2 is identified as the third gene with mutations found to be associated with a rare, inherited form of Alzheimer's disease.

1993: The Food and Drug Administration (FDA) approves the first Alzheimer's drug, tacrine (its brand name is Cognex). The drug targeted memory loss, among other dementia symptoms. Tacrine was eventually taken off the U.S. market in 2012 due to concerns regarding potential liver damage. Today, there are a total of five drugs approved to treat Alzheimer's. Chapter 5 discusses these drugs as well as other interventions and therapies used to treat the disease.

1993: Researchers identify APOE ε4, a form of the apolipoprotein E (APOE) gene on chromosome 19, as the first gene variation that increases an individual's risk for Alzheimer's. However, just because a person has this variation of the gene does not mean the person will definitely develop the disease. Chapter 3 discusses various risk factors of Alzheimer's.

1994: Former president of the United States Ronald Reagan announces that he has been diagnosed with Alzheimer's disease. In a letter to the American people about his decision to share his diagnosis, President Reagan writes that he hopes his letter may promote greater awareness of Alzheimer's, similar to when his wife Nancy had breast cancer. (Their disclosure of her cancer promoted more people to undergo cancer screening, which likely saved lives.) His letter does lead to greater awareness of the disease.

1994: The first World Alzheimer's Day (WAD) is established on September 21 by Alzheimer's Disease International. On World Alzheimer's Day, Alzheimer's organizations around the world concentrate their efforts on raising awareness about Alzheimer's and challenge the stigma that is associated with the disease and other dementias.

1995: Psychiatrists rediscover Auguste Deter's medical records in the archives at the University of Frankfurt. The 32-page file contains her admission report as well as three versions of the case history, including handwritten notes by Alzheimer.

1995: Researchers announce the first transgenic mouse model that develops Alzheimer-like brain pathology. The mouse is developed by inserting one of the human APP genes linked to a rare, inherited form of Alzheimer's disease.

1999: The first in a series of studies showing that injecting beta-amyloid into transgenic "Alzheimer" mice prevents plaques and other Alzheimer's-like brain changes is released.

2003: The National Alzheimer's Disease Genetics Study begins. Blood samples are collected from families with several members who developed Alzheimer's disease late in life in order to hopefully identify additional risk genes for the disease.

2004: The Alzheimer's Disease Neuroimaging Initiative (ADNI) study begins. Its goals are to determine whether standardized images, possibly combined with laboratory and psychological tests, can identify individuals who are at high risk for developing the disease, provide early detection, and monitor the effectiveness of treatment.

2006: The European Alzheimer's Disease Neuroimaging Initiative (E-ADNI) is launched. This initiative combines data from several European brain-imaging initiatives with ADNI data. This initiative is now worldwide. The World Wide ADNI (WW-ADNI) is a global network of research sites working together to improve diagnosis and speed up the development of treatment options.

2008: The Alzheimer's Association and the U.S. Centers for Disease Control and Prevention (CDC) launch the Healthy Brain Initiative with the publication of *A National Public Health Road Map to Maintaining Cognitive Health*. The goal of this initiative is to maintain or improve the cognitive performance of all adults (see "Directory of Resources"). In that same year, to further the work of global Alzheimer's research, the Alzheimer's Association creates the International Society to Advance Alzheimer's Research and Treatment (ISTAART), the first and only professional society dedicated to Alzheimer's and dementia.

2010: Alzheimer's becomes the sixth-leading cause of death in the United States. In this same year, a database is launched of 4,000 patients with Alzheimer's disease who participate in 11 pharmaceutical industry–sponsored clinical trials of Alzheimer's treatments. Data of this magnitude offer an unprecedented ability to understand the course of the disease.

2011: President Barack Obama signs the National Alzheimer's Project Act, which provides a national framework for a strategic plan to address the Alzheimer's crisis and coordinate research efforts. In this same year, a committee of experts review decades of previous research and find biomarker and neuroimaging evidence to warrant a change in how the disease is defined. It is determined that Alzheimer's disease should no longer be understood as simply a clinical syndrome of dementia but instead as a pathological process that develops into a clinical disease over the course of decades.

2013: Researchers working on the International Genomics of Alzheimer's Project (IGAP), identify 20 genetic variations associated with an increased risk of developing the disease.

2015: The Alzheimer's Accountability Act signed into law. The Alzheimer's Accountability Act ensures Congress hears directly from scientists. This law allows scientists at the NIH to directly send an annual research budget to Congress, bypassing the typical bureaucratic budget processes.

2018: President Trump signs into law a bill that allocates a historic $2.34 billion to Alzheimer's research funding for fiscal year 2019.

2021: The FDA approves a new medication to treat Alzheimer's. Under the accelerated approval pathway, Aducanumab (Aduhelm) is the first drug which may slow the progression of cognitive decline.

Alois Alzheimer thought what he found was a relatively rare disorder, but today we recognize Alzheimer's disease as the most common cause of the loss of mental function in people over the age of 65. As many as 5.8 million people in the United States have the disease. Given our aging population, it has been estimated that 14 million Americans will have Alzheimer's disease by the middle of this century unless we find a cure or ways to prevent the disease from developing. The next chapter discusses the onset of the disease as well as various causes and risk factors of Alzheimer's.

3

Causes and Risk Factors

Scientists believe that many factors influence when Alzheimer's disease begins and how it progresses. In most people, Alzheimer's results from a combination of genetic and environmental causes. Increasing age is the most important known risk factor for Alzheimer's. Scientists are working to understand how age-related changes in the brain can harm nerve cells and lead to the disease. Shrinkage of some areas of the brain, inflammation, the formation of unstable molecules called free radicals, and the breakdown of energy production within cells are all examples of age-related changes. Scientists have also learned that genes also play an important role in this disease. This chapter focuses on the causes and risk factors of Alzheimer's.

EARLY VERSUS LATE ONSET

There are two basic types of Alzheimer's disease: early-onset Alzheimer's disease and late-onset Alzheimer's disease. Early-onset Alzheimer's is a rare, predominantly inherited form of the disease. Early-onset Alzheimer's disease typically starts when people are in their 40s and 50s and represents less than 10% of all people with Alzheimer's. Some cases are caused by an inherited change in one of three genes, resulting in a type known as early-onset familial Alzheimer's disease, or EOFAD. A person whose biological mother or father bears the early-onset FAD genetic mutation has a fifty-fifty risk of inheriting it. If the mutation is hereditary, the child has a very high chance of developing early-onset FAD. Early-onset FAD is caused by a variety of single-gene mutations on chromosomes 21, 14, and 1. Each of these mutations results in the formation of abnormal proteins. Mutations on chromosome 21 result in the development of irregular amyloid precursor protein (APP), a protein whose exact function is not yet fully known. This breakdown is part of a mechanism that leads to the formation of toxic amyloid plaques, which are a characteristic of Alzheimer's disease. APP will be discussed later in this chapter when we examine the causes of Alzheimer's. A mutation on chromosome 14 results in the production of abnormal presenilin 1, while a mutation on chromosome 1 results in the production of abnormal presenilin 2. Presenilin is so named because a mutation in it triggers an aggressive, presenile type of Alzheimer's disease in people as early as in their 30s. Other cases of early-onset Alzheimer's disease may have a genetic component linked to factors other than these three genes, according to studies. Critical research findings regarding early-onset Alzheimer's have aided in the identification of crucial steps in the development of brain anomalies that are characteristic of the more common late-onset type of Alzheimer's. Genetics studies have helped explain why the disease develops in people at various ages.

Many experts believe that prior studies of potentially disease-modifying drugs in Alzheimer's disease have failed because the drugs were given too late in the disease's progression. As a result, many scientists have concentrated on explaining the mechanisms underlying preclinical Alzheimer's disease, which occurs when the brain pathology of Alzheimer's is present but not yet severe enough to cause symptoms. There are two large programs currently studying early-onset Alzheimer's: the Dominantly Inherited Alzheimer Network (DIAN) and the Alzheimer's Prevention Initiative. DIAN is a global database of people who are at risk of having autosomal-dominant Alzheimer's disease. The study's main goals are to look into the ordering of Alzheimer's pathophysiological changes in people who carry the mutations for the disease but have yet to show symptoms, and to find markers that signal the transition from normal cognitive functioning to symptoms of the disease. Scientists aim to gain insight into how and why Alzheimer's disease occurs in both its early- and late-onset manifestations by studying Alzheimer's-related brain changes that arise in these families well before signs of memory loss or cognitive problems emerge. The Alzheimer's Prevention Initiative is studying an extended family of 5,000 in Antioquia, Colombia, in which the disorder is present. Using brain imaging, cerebrospinal fluid (CSF), and cognitive outcomes, this initiative evaluates investigational amyloid-modifying treatments in healthy people who, based on their age and genetic background, are at the highest risk of developing EOFAD.

Alzheimer's early onset is uncommon. Most people with Alzheimer's have a late-onset form of the disease that usually reveals symptoms starting at the age of 65 or later. The causes of Alzheimer's late onset are yet to be fully understood; however, a combination of genetic, environmental, and lifestyle factors may be associated with a person's risk of disease. Any of these factors may differ from person to person in their importance for increasing or decreasing the risk of development. Researchers have yet to find a specific gene that directly causes the late-onset form of the disease. However, one genetic risk factor is having one form of the apolipoprotein E (APOE) gene on chromosome 19. APOE will be discussed further in this chapter when we examine the risk factors of Alzheimer's. In a review in 2016 in the journal *Genetics in Medicine*, the authors discussed using a relatively new approach called a genome-wide association study (GWAS), where researchers identify certain areas of genome (an organism's complete set of DNA, including all its genes) concern. By 2015, 33 areas of interest in the Alzheimer's genome had been confirmed. The complete DNA sequence of a person's genome is measured at once by a process called whole genome sequence. An additional method called entire exome sequencing examines the parts of the genome that code the protein directly. Researchers may find new genes that contribute to or defend against disease risk using these two methods. Recent findings have also revealed new information about the biological mechanisms involved in Alzheimer's disease, which may contribute to better treatments in the future.

CAUSES

Heredity

Each human cell has the instructions it requires to perform its function. DNA (deoxyribonucleic acid) is a molecule that contains these genetic instructions. DNA segments are called genes. Most humans have approximately 20,000 to 25,000 genes. People inherit two copies of each gene, one from their biological mother and the other from their biological father. Genes instruct the cell to produce specific proteins, which in turn determine the types of cells produced. Genes often control nearly every aspect of a cell's growth, function, and repair. For example, genes contain information that determines an individual's eye color, hair color, and whether they have cheek dimples. Genes also play a part in the health of the body's cells. Even minor variations in a gene can lead to diseases such as Alzheimer's.

A genetic mutation, or a permanent alteration in one or more particular genes, causes certain diseases. A person who inherits a genetic mutation that causes a particular disease from a biological parent is likely to develop that disease. Inherited genetic disorders include sickle cell anemia, cystic fibrosis, and EOFAD. In other diseases, a genetic variation may occur. Many variations may exist in a single gene. Sometimes, a variation in a gene can directly cause a disease. However, variations in genes are more likely to play a role in increasing or decreasing a person's likelihood of developing a disease rather than cause it directly. When a genetic variation increases the risk of developing a disease but does not directly cause it, it is known as a genetic risk factor. Regarding Alzheimer's, the earlier the onset of the disease, the greater the likelihood of a genetic cause. The likelihood of a genetic cause is greatest if the onset is before the age of 50 and lowest after the age of 70. A family history of early-onset Alzheimer's increases the likelihood of a genetic cause as well.

As mentioned earlier, FAD is a form of Alzheimer's disease that physicians know to be linked to genes. In families with FAD, at least two generations of members have had the disease. FAD accounts for less than 1% of all Alzheimer's cases, according to the National Institute on Aging (NIA). FAD is seen in the majority of people with early-onset Alzheimer's disease. One-quarter of all Alzheimer's disease cases are familial (i.e., three or more members of a family have the disease), while the other three-quarters are nonfamilial (i.e., an individual with Alzheimer's and no known family history of the disease). Since FAD and nonfamilial Alzheimer's disease tend to have the same clinical and pathologic phenotypes, family background and/or genetic testing are the only ways to tell them apart.

Senile Plaques and Neurofibrillary Tangles

Plaques and tangles are two of the most common signs of Alzheimer's disease. A senile plaque is a clump of protein that collects outside the cell. Beta-amyloid is the name for this protein. It is a fragment of APP. These protein fragments are broken down and removed in a healthy brain. In Alzheimer's disease, the fragments clump together to form rigid, plaques. Dale Bredesen and other researchers at the Buck Institute for Research on Aging, in Novato, California, have studied beta-amyloid in mice. They discovered that blocking particular events inside neurons can prevent memory problems in mice even though the mice have a lot of plaques. The beta-amyloid peptide, which forms plaques in Alzheimer's, is a major issue. According to the Alzheimer's Association, beta-amyloid is chemically "stickier" than other fragments that are produced when APP is cut. It builds up in stages: the pieces first form small clusters known as oligomers, then chain of clusters known as fibrils, and finally "mats" of fibrils known as beta-sheets. Plaques, which consist of clumps of beta-sheets and other substances, are the final stage.

Twisted fibers within the brain's cells are known as neurofibrillary tangles. Tau protein is the main component of these tangles. Tau forms part of a structure in a neuron called a microtubule. The microtubule aids in the transportation of nutrients and other essential substances from one part of the neuron to another. However, in Alzheimer's disease, the tau protein is irregular, and the microtubule structures collapse and form the tangles. The role tau plays in Alzheimer's will be further discussed later in this chapter.

APP

A healthy adult brain has about 100 billion neurons (i.e., nerve cells), each with long, branch-like extensions called dendrites. Dendrites enable neurons to form connections with one another. At such connections, called synapses (or tiny gaps), information flows in tiny bursts of chemicals called neurotransmitters, which are released by the axon terminal of one neuron and detected by the dendrites of another neuron. There are approximately 100 trillion synapses in the brain. These tiny gaps allow signals to pass quickly through neuronal circuits in the brain, forming the cellular foundation for everything from our sensations and feelings to our thoughts and movements.

In the brain, APP is thought to be responsible for forming and repairing synapses. In its complete form, APP extends from the inside of brain cells to the outside by passing through the fatty membrane around the cell. As a result, a portion of APP resides in the wall of a cell, and a portion of it sticks out of the cell. When APP is activated, there is a cut: the protein separates, and part is released from the cell. If APP activation causes only one cut, called a singlet, it is fine: that happens to everyone. If APP activation causes more than a few cuts, the parts find each other and become doublets, triplets, or quadruplets, and that is what causes problems in the brain. Two enzymes cut this protein in an organized manner: one is beta secretase, which cuts at the beginning, and the other is gamma secretase, which cuts at the end. If people have too much activity by beta secretase, then they make too much amyloid beta and it builds up. If people have too much activity at the second cut, gamma secretase, they are also at risk for Alzheimer's. Other people with Alzheimer's cut the protein at a typical rate, but their problem is one of removal: they have a problem with removing the amyloid-beta peptide from the brain. The APOE ε4 gene is known to be responsible for removal. People with the APOE ε4 gene are at a greater risk of developing Alzheimer's disease. The APOE ε4 gene as a risk factor will be discussed later in this chapter.

Researchers at the Buck Institute have also discovered the role that peptide C31 may play in Alzheimer's. C31, which is released within neurons, is one of the peptides cut from APP. C31, the researchers reasoned, could alter signaling patterns in neurons, causing them to die. To test their hypothesis, they created a change in the APP gene that prevents C31 from being released. In a mouse model of Alzheimer's disease, the mutation they introduced did indeed prevent C31 from being cut by APP. The researchers discovered that these mice produced a lot of plaques but did not have any memory issues. Nor was there any synapse damage or brain atrophy in the mice. These researchers at Buck believe that while beta-amyloid causes plaques to develop on the outside of the cell, the disease process requires C31 to be released within the cell to trigger cell destruction. Scientists are now looking for drugs that can prevent C31 from being cut. Even if excess beta-amyloid in a person's brain cannot be removed, Alzheimer's memory loss can be avoided if researchers can develop a treatment that prevents C31 from being cut by APP.

Tau

Scientists have long emphasized the significance of tau in Alzheimer's disease due to evidence linking the spread of tau with disease progression. As previously mentioned, a likely cause of Alzheimer's is the accumulation of the protein fragment beta-amyloid, which occurs outside neurons. Tau is a small protein contained within the axons of neurons. It helps form microtubules, essential structures that transport nutrients within neurons. Among tau's multiple functions in healthy brain cells, a very important one is stabilization of the internal microtubules that cells use to distribute nutrients and other important substances from one part of a neuron to another. In individuals with Alzheimer's, an abnormal form of tau accumulates inside neurons. Even before it gathers, malfunctioning tau can damage cellular transportation by blocking the microtubule tracks. Beta-amyloid plaques cause neurons to die by interfering with them communicating with one another, while clumps of tau block the transport of nutrients and other essential molecules inside neurons. Tau accumulation tends to begin in the parts of the brain called the hippocampus and entorhinal cortex which are involved in the formation and processing of memories, and it continues to accumulate in other areas of the brain as the disease progresses.

Besides the microtubular form, which is composed of many tau molecules, tau also exists in smaller versions, called oligomers, which are made up of fewer tau proteins. Recent evidence suggests that tau spreads through the brain by means of oligomer "seeds" that travel across synapses from one neuron to the dendrite of another neuron. Tau in smaller forms circulates within neurons, disrupting cellular function. These formations are discovered in the brains of people who are developing Alzheimer's disease decades before the disease manifests clinically. The amount of abnormal tau in the brain is related to the stage of the disease, with individuals in later stages having more abnormal amounts of tau than individuals in early stages of the disease.

Decrease in Acetylcholine

Among those who study the pathology of Alzheimer's disease, the focus tends to be on the plaques and the tangles. However, another significant finding had arisen before researchers started to investigate the molecular foundations of plaques and tangles. This finding involved a neurotransmitter called acetylcholine (ACh). Some neurons in the brain that use ACh seem to be more impaired than others; they are said to show a cholinergic deficit. The cholinergic deficit discovered in Alzheimer's disease stems from early research that found that cholinergic neurons that project from lower brain areas up to higher brain areas involved in memory are lost early in the disease progression. This discovery prompted scientists to look for ways to boost ACh levels or defend these neurons in some way. One such way is through a drug called donepezil, commonly referred to as Aricept. Aricept is a cholinesterase inhibitor. It prevents the breakdown of ACh so that it stays around longer. For a long time, many of the treatments for individuals living with Alzheimer's were aimed at replacing the missing ACh. Current research is attempting to progress toward drugs that modify the disease, that is, toward drugs that would have a significant impact on the disease's origin, the plaques and tangles. Chapter 5 discusses cholinesterase inhibitors and other pharmacological treatments in greater detail.

Defective Genes

The approximately 20,000 to 25,000 genes that each person possesses present many situations where something can go wrong. Several genetic associations with Alzheimer's disease have been discovered, including C9ORF72, TOMM40, and TREM2. People with both early- and late-onset forms of the disease have been shown to have a mutated C9ORF72 gene. This gene produces a protein that controls intracellular matrix transportation. The mutation was already known to play a role in ALS and frontotemporal dementia, but new research shows that it also interferes with a crucial DNA repair mechanism. Alzheimer's disease has a complicated relationship with the TOMM40 gene, which is a protein-coding gene. The impact of this gene depends on whether someone has a biological parent diagnosed with the disease. Individuals who have a parent with Alzheimer's and have a longer variation of the TOMM40 gene are more likely to develop dementia than those with its shorter genetic variant. However, individuals who have the longer variation of the TOMM40 gene but do not have a parent with Alzheimer's have better memory than those with the shorter genetic variant. This implies that the effect of the variation of the TOMM40 gene depends on family history of the disease. Normally, TREM2 (triggering receptor expressed on myeloid cells-2) protein helps regulate removal of cell debris, clearing amyloid proteins and suppressing inflammation in microglia. Researchers noted in a 2018 review in the journal *Molecular Neurodegeneration* that with the TREM2 gene, loss-of-function mutations cause a sequence of physiological events associated with Alzheimer's disease. The findings indicate that TREM2 plays a significant role in Alzheimer's disease at the level of amyloid and tau pathologies, as well as inflammation, either alone or in combination with other molecules such as APOE. Studies focusing on TREM2 in the context of Alzheimer's illustrate its complexity. TREM2 may be harmful in the early stages of the disease and then become beneficial in the later stages of the disease.

RISK FACTORS

Advanced Age

Increasing age is the most important known risk factor for Alzheimer's. The number of people with the disease doubles every five years beyond age 65. About one-third of all people age 85 and older may have Alzheimer's disease. One of the great mysteries of Alzheimer's disease is that it mostly affects the elderly. This subject is being researched in the context of typical brain aging. Scientists are learning, for example, how age-related changes in the brain can harm neurons and affect other types of brain cells, resulting in Alzheimer's disease damage. Atrophy or shrinking of certain parts of the brain, inflammation, vascular damage, the formation of unstable molecules called free radicals, and mitochondrial dysfunction (a breakdown of energy production within a cell) are all examples of age-related changes. However, it is important to remember that Alzheimer's disease is not a typical part of aging, and that being older is not enough to cause the disease.

Family History

A family history of Alzheimer's is not necessary for an individual to develop the disease. However, individuals who have a first-degree biological relative (e.g., parent, brother, or sister) with Alzheimer's are more likely to develop the disease than those who do not have a close biological relative with the disease. Also, those who have more than one first-degree relative with Alzheimer's are at an even higher risk for developing the disease.

APOE ε4

The APOE gene directs the development of a protein known as apolipoprotein E. Lipoproteins are formed as this protein interacts with fats (i.e., lipids) in the body. Lipoproteins are responsible for transporting cholesterol and other fats through the bloodstream. Maintaining normal cholesterol levels is important for the prevention of cardiovascular diseases, such as heart attack and stroke. The APOE gene is found on chromosome 19 and comes in several different variations called alleles (e.g., APOE ε2, APOE ε3, APOE ε4). Each person receives two alleles of a gene, one from each biological parent. This combination is one factor among many that influence a variety of processes in the body.

Researchers studying APOE at autopsy have found that APOE ε2 is relatively rare and appears to provide some protection against the disease. If Alzheimer's disease occurs in a person with this allele, it usually develops later in life than it would in someone with the APOE ε4 gene. APOE ε3 is the most common allele, found in more than half of the general population. It is believed to play a neutral role in the disease; which means that having this form neither increases nor decreases one's risk of developing the disease. APOE ε4 increases risk for Alzheimer's disease and is also associated with an earlier age of disease onset. A person has zero, one, or two APOE ε4 alleles. Those who inherit one copy of the APOE ε4 allele have an increased chance of developing the disease, and those who inherit two copies have an even higher risk. For example, Jing Qian and colleagues, in 2017, determined that people who have one copy of the APOE ε4 allele have approximately a 10% to 20% chance of developing Alzheimer's by age 75, whereas people who have two copies have about a 25% to 35% risk. When compared to people with Alzheimer's disease who do not have this variation, the APOE ε4 allele can be linked to an early occurrence of memory loss and other symptoms. The relationship between the APOE ε4 allele and the risk of Alzheimer's disease is unknown. However, researchers discovered that this allele is linked to an increased number of amyloid plaques in affected people's brain tissue. APOE ε4 binds to beta-amyloid quickly, which may lead to disproportionate amounts in the brain. As discussed earlier in this chapter, buildup of amyloid plaques may lead to the death of neurons and the progressive signs and symptoms of this disorder.

It is important to note that APOE ε4 is called a risk factor gene because it increases a person's risk of developing the disease. However, inheriting an APOE ε4 allele does not mean that a person will definitely develop Alzheimer's. Some people with an APOE ε4 allele never get the disease, and others who develop Alzheimer's do not have any APOE ε4 alleles. For instance, it is estimated that 42% of persons with Alzheimer's do not have an APOE ε4 allele.

Vascular and Metabolic Conditions

The health of our heart and blood vessels has an effect on our brain health. Although the brain accounts for just 2% of our body weight, it uses 20% of our body's energy and oxygen. A healthy heart pumps enough blood to the brain, while healthy blood vessels allow oxygen and nutrient-rich blood to enter the brain in order for it to function properly. Therefore, it should be no surprise that researchers are investigating whether vascular and metabolic conditions play a role in the development and progression of Alzheimer's disease. For instance, scientists are investigating the relationship between cognitive decline and vascular conditions, such as heart disease, stroke, and hypertension, as well as metabolic conditions, such as diabetes and obesity. Many factors that increase the risk of cardiovascular disease are also associated with a higher risk of developing dementia. For instance, some research suggests impaired glucose processing, which is a precursor to diabetes, may increase the risk of developing dementia. Similarly, middle-aged adults who are dealing with hypertension, high cholesterol, and obesity are at an increased risk of developing dementia. Building on the connection between heart health and brain health, researchers have discovered that factors that protect the heart may also protect the brain and reduce the risk of developing Alzheimer's or other dementias. Physical activity appears to be one of these factors. Chapter 8 discusses the role exercise plays in reducing one's risk of developing Alzheimer's disease.

Lifestyle

As mentioned, engaging in physical activity appears to minimize the risk of someone developing Alzheimer's or some other dementia. Although researchers have studied a wide variety of exercises, they do not yet know which specific types of exercise may be most effective in reducing risk; however, they recently discovered that frequency and intensity matter. The more often people exercise and the more strenuous the exercise, the more likely they are to reduce their risk of Alzheimer's (see chapter 8). In addition to physical activity, new research indicates that eating a heart-healthy diet is linked to a lower risk of developing dementia. Fruits, vegetables, whole grains, fish, chicken, nuts, and legumes are all important components of a heart-healthy diet. However, individuals should limit their intake of saturated fats, red meat, and sugar. Researchers have started looking at whether a combination of health factors and lifestyle habits (such as blood pressure and physical activity) can better predict Alzheimer's and dementia risk than individual risk factors.

Additionally, studies suggest that remaining socially and mentally active throughout life and how we handle stress may support brain health and possibly reduce the risk of Alzheimer's and other dementias. These researchers used data gathered from the Health and Retirement Study, a large, nationally representative population of over 16,000 American adults age 50 and older who were followed prospectively for six years. Ertel and colleagues examined whether social integration, which is how well incorporated people are to and within their social group, predicted memory change. The researchers measured social integration based on marital status, volunteer activities, and frequency of contact with children, parents, and neighbors. Participants took memory tests at two-year intervals during the course of the six years. Researchers read a list of 10 common nouns to survey respondents, who were then asked to recall as many words as possible immediately and again after a five-minute delay. It was found that individuals in their 50s and 60s who had high levels of social integration also had the slowest rate of memory decline. Participants with the highest social integration ratings had less than half the rate of memory loss as compared to those who were the least socially involved. Additionally, individuals with the least years of formal schooling seemed to benefit the most from an active social life as they grew older. Overall, the results from this study suggest that increasing social integration may be an important component of efforts to protect older adults from memory decline. More research is needed to better understand how social and cognitive engagement may affect biological processes to reduce risk. Physical activity, a nutritious diet, and social engagement have been associated with helping people stay healthy as they age. Research indicates these lifestyle factors may also help reduce the risk of cognitive decline and of developing Alzheimer's disease. Lifestyle factors will be further discussed in chapter 8.

Education Level

People with more years of formal education are at lower risk for Alzheimer's and other dementias than those with fewer years of formal education. Some researchers believe that having more years of education builds "cognitive reserve." Cognitive reserve refers to the brain's ability to make flexible and efficient use of its cognitive resources. In other words, it is the brain's ability to adapt and get the job done in spite of challenges. The number of years of formal education is not the only determinant of cognitive reserve. Having a mentally stimulating job and engaging in other mentally stimulating activities may also help build cognitive reserve. As mentioned previously, remaining socially and mentally active is important with regard to memory and the idea of cognitive reserve, but the exact mechanism by which this may occur is unknown.

As discussed in chapter 1, there are racial/ethnic differences in prevalence rates regarding Alzheimer's. But socioeconomic characteristics, including lower levels of education and higher rates of poverty, and not genetic factors are the most likely reasons why older Black/African Americans and Hispanics are more likely, on a per capita basis, than older whites to develop Alzheimer's or other dementias. Dr. Jennifer Manly, a neuropsychologist, looked at how cultural interactions, especially the quality of early education, influence people's brains as they grow older. Dr. Manly found that the majority of African Americans she interviewed attended segregated schools in the South, many of which were located in rural areas. Her research revealed that the duration of the school year, the amount of money spent on each student, and the student-teacher ratio had an effect on older people's performance on memory, executive function, and language tests, regardless of race. She found no difference in the rate of cognitive loss when she compared the outcomes of memory tests in African Americans and white Americans who had obtained the same quality of education. This tells us that school quality is likely a factor related to cognitive impairment.

TBI and CTE

Traumatic brain injury (TBI) is the disruption of normal brain function caused by a blow or jolt to the head or the penetration of the skull by a foreign object. The leading causes of TBI that have resulted in emergency department visits, according to the Centers for Disease Control and Prevention (CDC), were falls, being hit by an object, and motor vehicle accidents. TBI increases the risk of developing Alzheimer's or some other form of dementia. The number of TBIs sustained increases the risk of dementia.

People who have had even a mild TBI have a higher risk of dementia than those who have not had a TBI.

Chronic traumatic encephalopathy (CTE) is also linked to the development of dementia. CTE is associated with repeated blows to the head, such as those that may occur while playing contact sports. CTE is a neuropathologic diagnosis, meaning it is characterized by brain changes that can only be identified during an autopsy. Currently, there is no test to determine if someone has brain changes due to CTE while the person is alive. Similar to Alzheimer's disease, CTE is characterized by tangles of an abnormal form of the protein tau in the brain. Unlike Alzheimer's disease, these tangles typically appear around small blood vessels, and beta-amyloid plaques are not commonly present. How the brain changes associated with CTE are linked to cognitive or behavioral dysfunction is not yet clear. What is clear is that trauma to the brain increases one's risk of developing Alzheimer's or another dementia.

At the beginning of this chapter, we noted increasing age as the most important known risk factor for Alzheimer's. However, as the rest of the chapter illustrates, Alzheimer's is complex. There are many different causes and risk factors that contribute to the development of the disease. Scientists are conducting studies to learn more about the biological characteristics as well as environmental factors that contribute to Alzheimer's disease. Findings from these studies will help better understand the causes of Alzheimer's and make diagnosis easier. The next chapter focuses on the warning signs and symptoms of Alzheimer's.

4

Signs and Symptoms

The first symptoms of Alzheimer's vary from person to person. For many people, decline in certain aspects of their cognitive abilities, such as word finding, visual/spatial problems, and impaired thought or judgment, may signs of Alzheimer's disease in its early stages. Alzheimer's disease causes changes in the brain that begin years before symptoms appear. *Preclinical* Alzheimer's disease refers to this time span (see chapter 6). Alzheimer's disease symptoms will worsen over time, but the pace at which the disease progresses will vary. On average, a person with Alzheimer's lives 4 to 8 years after diagnosis but can live as long as 20 years, depending on other factors.

Individuals with Alzheimer's disease will function independently in the early/mild stage. Many continue to drive, work, and participate in a variety of social activities. Despite this, the individual can experience memory problems, such as forgetting familiar words or where everyday items are located. Family and close friends often begin to notice these changes. The middle/moderate stage of Alzheimer's is typically the longest; it can last for many years. During the moderate stage of Alzheimer's, the symptoms are more pronounced. A person may take longer in or have difficulty with performing everyday tasks, such as getting dressed, handling money, or paying bills. During this stage, individuals may still remember significant details about their life; however, some have trouble recognizing family and friends. They can start to mix up words, become irritated or angry, or behave in unusual ways, such as refusing to take a shower. Damage to brain nerve cells may make it difficult for them to articulate thoughts and carry out these simple tasks. Other symptoms during this stage often include wandering or getting lost, repeating questions, and misplacing things or leaving objects in unusual places, as well as personality and behavior changes, such as hallucinations, delusions, paranoia, and/or impulsive behavior. The person with Alzheimer's disease will need more treatment as the disease progresses. Individuals who are in the late/severe stage of the disease lose their ability to react to their surroundings, carry on a conversation, and, finally, regulate movement. They are completely dependent on others for care as their body begins shutting down. They may still be able to say words or phrases, but eventually their speech gradually becomes reduced to groans, moans, and grunts. During this time, they become increasingly sleepy and finally bedridden. Weight loss, seizures, trouble swallowing, skin infections, and a lack of bowel and bladder control are among their other possible symptoms. Alzheimer's disease is ultimately fatal. As a result of the body shutting down, aspiration pneumonia is a common cause of death in people with Alzheimer's disease. It occurs when a person can no longer swallow properly, resulting in food or liquids entering the lungs (see chapter 6 for a detailed discussion of the stages of Alzheimer's).

Researchers are currently investigating biomarkers that are biological indicators of disease present in brain images, cerebrospinal fluid (CSF), and blood to identify early changes in the brains of people with mild cognitive impairment (MCI; see below) and cognitively normal people who may be at higher risk for Alzheimer's disease, as described in chapter 2. While studies suggest that such early detection is feasible, further research is required before these techniques can be widely used in ordinary medical practice to diagnose Alzheimer's disease (see chapter 5 for more information on biomarkers).

This chapter focuses on the major warning signs and symptoms of the disease as compared to typical age-related changes in function. Keep in mind, individuals may encounter one or more of these warning signs to different degrees, and they do need to experience every warning sign or symptom for you to be worried about them.

GRADUAL MEMORY LOSS

Have you ever forgotten where you parked your car, misplaced your house keys, or walked into a room and forgot why you went in there? This has happened to everyone at one time or another and are examples of typical age-related forgetfulness. Most memory issues associated with age are not symptoms of dementia or Alzheimer's disease but rather evidence of a slowdown in the brain's processing speed, which lengthens the time it takes us to retrieve information. When we get older, our capacity to split our focus deteriorates, which can make it difficult to store new memories. The signs of Alzheimer's are different from these kinds of typical age-related memory issues.

According to the Alzheimer's Association, memory problems are often one of the first signs of cognitive dysfunction associated with Alzheimer's disease. At first, only short-term memory may be affected, such as forgetting recently learned information, with long-term memory issues developing later. People may forget an appointment or the name of someone they recently met. Many people complain about memory loss, yet they may describe cases of forgetfulness in great detail, including where they were at the time. Other memory issues involve missing important dates or events, repeatedly asking for the same information, and a growing need to rely on external memory aids (e.g., reminder memos or electronic devices) or family members for tasks that were previously done independently.

For some people with memory problems, MCI may be the issue. People with MCI have more memory issues than other people their age may have, but their symptoms do not interfere with their daily lives. They can still look after themselves and go about their daily routines. Memory issues associated with MCI include often misplacing belongings, failing to attend activities or appointments, and having more difficulty coming up with words than other people of a similar age. Issues with movement and problems involving the sense of smell have also been attributed to MCI. It can be an early sign of Alzheimer's. However, not everyone with MCI will develop Alzheimer's disease. Even though Alzheimer's disease is more common in older adults with MCI, it does not affect everyone. Some may even go back to normal cognitive function.

How do these memory issues differ from typical age-related changes in cognition? Recall that not remembering where you parked your car in a parking garage, or losing something and then remembering where you left is going to happen to most people. As we get older, our brain takes longer to process information, we are more easily distracted, and we have more trouble dividing our attention between two different tasks.

DECLINE IN ABILITY TO PERFROM ROUTINE TASKS

Maybe your memory seems fine, but keeping track of monthly bills and managing your home finances have become much more difficult. Or you have always been known for your great cooking, but lately the multiple steps in familiar recipes do not seem to make sense anymore. Some people's ability to create and execute a strategy, as well as their ability to deal with numbers, deteriorates. They can find it difficult to concentrate and take much longer to complete tasks than before. People living with Alzheimer's often find it hard to complete daily tasks. Simple tasks that were once simple can become much more difficult. They can have difficulty driving to a familiar place, handling a work budget, forgetting how to prepare a simple meal, or recalling the rules of a favorite game. Forgetting how to use the stove or oven, to lock the house when leaving, or to get dressed can also be signs of Alzheimer's disease. It is important to note that this is not an effort to learn something different, such as a new computer program, but rather a shift in their ability to accomplish a job they have always been able to do until recently. Typical age-related changes include sometimes requiring assistance with microwave settings, recording a television program, using a new television remote, or making an occasional error when balancing a checkbook.

IMPAIRMENT OF JUDGMENT

People with Alzheimer's may experience changes in judgment or decision-making. Impairment of judgment refers to the inability to make appropriate decisions. Someone who has Alzheimer's disease or another form of dementia may be unable to assess the various factors that should be considered when making a decision. In Alzheimer's disease, poor judgment is more than just one bad decision; it is a series of unmistakably incorrect decisions or behavior. Here are a couple of examples of poor judgment illustrated by individuals living with Alzheimer's disease. They may make poor financial decisions, such as contributing large sums to telemarketers or giving money away carelessly. Some individuals living with Alzheimer's are less concerned with hygiene or keeping themselves clean. For instance, there may be a sudden decrease in how often they bathe themselves, a desire to wear the same clothes for many days in a row without washing them, or a lack of judgment in terms of being appropriately dressed for the weather. A typical age-related change is making a bad decision or mistake once in a while.

DISORIENTATION

Most people know what it is like to be driving and momentarily forget where they were going. Getting lost in one's own neighborhood or losing track of the day or time, on the other hand, may be symptoms of dementia or Alzheimer's disease. People with Alzheimer's often get confused with time or place. Dates, seasons, and even the passing of time can be lost on them. For example, as Alzheimer's disease progresses, it is not uncommon for these individuals to think they are several years younger than they are, due to their unawareness of time passing.

People living with Alzheimer's often misplace things and lose the ability to retrace their steps. They may put things in unusual places; for example, they may put their eyeglasses in the refrigerator. They will likely not only lose items but also find it all the more difficult to retrace their steps to find the objects. Since "someone" placed their eyeglasses in the refrigerator or "took" their wallet, individuals with dementia may become irritated. They cannot find their keys, but they have no idea how the keys ended up in the cabinet. This may lead them to suspect others of stealing on occasion, and this suspiciousness can become more common over time.

Due to problems with short-term memory, they may have difficulty understanding something if it does not happen right away. Sometimes they lose track of where they are or how they got to that location. They may wander away from the house and forget how to get home, or they may not able to assess traffic in order to decide whether it is safe to cross the street at that moment. As a result, they do not recognize the danger of walking across a busy street during rush-hour traffic. Misplacing items occasionally and needing to retrace one's steps are common age-related changes, as is being confused about the day of the week but eventually figuring it out.

WITHDRAWAL

People with Alzheimer's may start to give up hobbies, social activities, or playing sports they previously enjoyed. They may have difficulty remembering how to finish something they have been working on—for example, knitting a hat—or have trouble following a favorite sports team. Because of the changes they experience, they may avoid social situations. They may, for example, not want to visit with cherished grandchildren, they abandon longtime hobbies, such as sewing or woodworking, or they forgo regular gatherings with friends. If they are still working, they may fail to complete work-related assignments or may miss several days of work at a time. This lack of interest and this withdrawal from people and activities around them can increase as symptoms worsen. A typical change as we get older is needing a longer break between activities or sometimes feeling tired from work, family, or social obligations.

MOOD OR PERSONALITY CHANGES

The mood and personalities of people with Alzheimer's can change. It is normal for people to slow down as they get older—they may not want to attend events with a large number of people if they have experienced a decline in their eyesight or hearing, or they may give up physically demanding activities. Changes in a person's basic personality or temperament, on the other hand, are not typical and could indicate Alzheimer's disease or some cognitive impairment. A person who was once outgoing and social may become withdrawn, or a person who was once cheerful may become obstinate, distrustful, frustrated, or sad. The person could become perplexed, suspicious, afraid, or anxious as a result. For example, the individual may say that someone who's offered to help clean the house just wants to steal money or other valuables from the house. Furthermore, when anything out of the ordinary occurs, the person may become increasingly agitated. For instance, Alzheimer's patients have been known to become extremely upset to find out a local store stopped carrying their favorite snack. They can also become easily troubled at home, at work, with friends, or in situations outside of their comfort zones. Depression often accompanies Alzheimer's disease, and symptoms include a loss of interest in a favorite activity, a change in appetite, changes in sleep—for example, difficulty falling asleep or sleeping too much—fatigue, and a feeling of hopelessness.

As we age, becoming a little more "set in our ways," irritable when a routine is disrupted and generally disliking of change are typical. If someone has always been temperamental or cranky, it is unlikely that this quality is related to the person's cognitive functioning. However, if there has been a change in the person's normal mood and actions over the last few months, it may be an indication of atypical changes in the brain.

These mood and personality changes can be very difficult to deal with; however, it is important to remember these changes are due to the disease. The individual is not purposely trying to annoy people or hurt their feelings. Try not to argue with the person; instead, focus on the feelings, not the words, that the person expresses. Instead of trying to negotiate with the individual, set fair standards and use redirection and diversion. If the personality change is abrupt, it may be helpful to consult a doctor to see if these sudden mood or personality changes are due to something else, such as delirium.

According to Esther Heerema, a licensed social worker who has worked with numerous individuals with Alzheimer's disease and other dementias, delirium is a disturbance in one's thinking. Its onset is sudden, and it typically has an external cause. One day, the person is doing fine, and the next day, the person may be very confused and unable to get dressed in the morning. Delirium is typically brought about by a specific illness, such as a urinary tract infection, pneumonia, dehydration, substance use, or drug or alcohol withdrawal. Medications that interfere with one another are the most common cause of delirium. The good news is that delirium is usually temporary if the underlying cause is detected and treated.

VISUAL/SPATIAL CHANGES

As we get older, we are at more risk for certain age-related visual complications such as cataracts (i.e., the clouding of the lens of the eye), glaucoma (i.e., condition in which a buildup of pressure causes damage to the optic nerve), or age-related macular degeneration (i.e., progressive degeneration of the macula, a small group of cells located in the retina that help produce central vision).

Nevertheless, for some people, having vision problems is a sign of Alzheimer's. They may have trouble measuring distance and distinguishing color or contrast, which can lead to driving issues. Because of changes in the ability to understand spatial relationships, driving can become more difficult as the disease progresses. Due to a loss in visual-spatial skills, navigating a turn, changing lanes, or parking a vehicle, for example, may become a major challenge. As the disease advances, it may become necessary to have a conversation about no longer driving. While this may be a tough subject to broach, if individuals are afraid to ride in the car while the person is driving, it is a pretty straightforward indication that the person should not be driving. Driving necessitates the use of various facets of the brain, and these abilities begin to deteriorate as Alzheimer's symptoms develop. If there are concerns about a loved one's continued ability to drive, you may want to have the person's driving ability evaluated through a test at a driving.

Not only can visual-spatial changes impact driving but they also can affect depth perception, making it more difficult to navigate tasks such as going up or down the stairs as well as getting in and out of bed, and thus increasing the risk of falls. Activities of daily living (ADLs), in other words, tasks that need to be accomplished on a regular basis to functions such as bathing, getting dressed, or eating can therefore become more challenging.

LOSS OF LANGUAGE SKILLS

Another symptom of Alzheimer's disease is having trouble with language and communication. People with Alzheimer's may stop in the middle of a conversation, be unsure how to proceed, or repeat themselves. They may struggle with vocabulary, have difficulty finding the right word or refer to items incorrectly (e.g., calling a watch a "hand clock"). In order to compensate, they may try describing an object rather than using a name for it—for example, referring to the telephone as "that thing I call people with." Keep in mind, as we age, we sometimes have trouble finding the right word for something; however, for individuals living with Alzheimer's, it is much more than that. Their challenges will render them unable to join a discussion or follow along with one. They will often repeat the same stories. Additionally, their ability to read or write may become impaired.

WHAT TO DO?

It can be difficult to know what to do if you find one or more of these warning signs or symptoms in yourself or one of your loved ones. It is natural to be hesitant or fearful of sharing these changes with others. However, these are serious health concerns that should be evaluated by a physician, and it is important to find out what is happening. The Alzheimer's Association advises that you open the conversation. If you recognize some of the warning signs in yourself, talk to someone you can trust about it. Similarly, if you detect memory changes in a family member or friend, determine who would be most appropriate to talk with the person. Once the determination is made, have the discussion as soon as possible, since early detection and treatment are important (see chapter 5 for diagnosis and treatment of the disease). Keep in mind that some people may dismiss your concerns because they attribute memory, perception, or behavior issues to stress or typical aging. Therefore, the first conversation may not be successful, so you may need to have more than one conversation. It may be helpful to take notes during the discussion to aid you in planning for the next conversation. Consider what worked well and what could be done differently next time.

Next, make an appointment to see a doctor. As discussed in chapter 1, a variety of conditions can produce cognitive changes, so it is important to have a complete medical examination to see whether the symptoms are linked to Alzheimer's disease or some other condition. For example, certain conditions can cause short-term or long-term memory loss and affect thinking or behavior. Additionally, cognitive and/or behavioral changes may be caused by environmental stressors, such as family discord, or by medical conditions, such as diabetes or depression. If the cause is not Alzheimer's or another dementia, it could be a treatable condition. If it is Alzheimer's or another dementia, getting a diagnosis early and accurately has many advantages, including the ability to prepare for the future, to access support services, and to access medication that can help manage cognitive, emotional, and behavioral symptoms. These and other steps will be examined in greater detail in chapter 7, when we discuss the effects Alzheimer's has on the family and friends of the person living with the disease.

Now that you have a better idea of the warning signs and symptoms of Alzheimer's, see the next chapter to focus on the diagnostic process and treatment of the disease.

5

Diagnosis, Treatment, and Management

There is no single test to determine if someone has Alzheimer's disease. In order to reach a diagnosis, physicians and other specialists use multiple evaluation methods and assessment technologies to determine if a dementia diagnosis is warranted. In most cases, diagnosing Alzheimer's disease begins with an office examination provided by a health-care professional. The evaluation will likely involve several components. The physician will likely begin by asking the patient (and family members, if they are present) to describe their current difficulties and the reasons that motivated them to seek treatment. The doctor will ask questions to gather more information and to clarify understanding of the issues presented by the patient/family. Doctors will typically conduct a physical examination to rule out other possible medical illnesses that could contribute to dementia-like symptoms and will also administer a mental-status exam (an interview protocol) in order to assess for cognitive, emotional, motor, and perpetual deficits. The next steps may involve ordering blood tests to gather additional information about organ health and conducting neuropsychological tests to more precisely assess cognitive functions such as memory, decision-making, problem-solving, and verbal ability. Brain-imaging scans are also part of the standard evaluation procedure and are used to detect evidence of tumors, stroke, or physical trauma. Typically, several office appointments are necessary for the clinician to gather sufficient data in order to make an informed decision about whether a patient meets the criteria for Alzheimer's disease or a related disorder.

ALZHEIMER'S DISEASE DIAGNOSIS

In order to accurately diagnose any medical or psychiatric condition, a clinician must carefully determine if a patient's symptoms are consistent with a standardized set of diagnostic criteria: specific signs, symptoms, and other requirements that must be met by the patient (and confirmed by a clinician) before a formal diagnosis is made. Classification systems provide formal listings of diagnostic labels (names of various disorders), their diagnostic criteria, and a diagnostic code used for categorization, data collection, and billing purposes.

Diagnostic Systems and Criteria

Several classification systems have been developed to define the diagnostic criteria for dementia, a class of neurological disorders marked by memory deficits. These diagnostic guidelines have undergone significant revision over the past decade, creating some potential confusion about the terminologies commonly used to describe Alzheimer's disease. Importantly, the American Psychiatric Association published the fifth edition of the *Diagnostic and Statistical Manual of Mental Disorders* (*DSM-5*) in 2013, which made significant changes to the diagnostic nomenclature for dementia. Importantly, this turn of the tide renamed dementia to "major neurocognitive disorder" in an effort to reduce the stigma associated with the older term. However, "dementia" is still used today as an acceptable alternative, and both labels describe essentially the same set of symptoms. The *DSM-5* also classifies earlier stages of cognitive decline as "mild neurocognitive disorder," which now allows for a diagnosis of less-disabling cognitive syndromes that are now believed to deserve significant clinical attention. This change in the diagnostic system reflects a modernized effort to diagnose neurocognitive disorders as early as possible so that intervention may take place during the frequently long preclinical period before major decline is present (see chapter 10). The diagnosis of "mild neurocognitive decline" is equivalent to "mild cognitive impairment" (MCI) and "prodromal dementia"—again, different labels are used to describe the same condition. Another commonly used classification system, the *International Classification of Diseases* (*ICD*), developed by the World Health Organization (WHO), saw an update in 2018 and adopted much of the same terminology used in the *DSM-5*, and it requires very similar diagnostic criteria. However, the *DSM*-5 mostly focuses on the classification and diagnosis of mental health disorders and is used almost exclusively in the United States, whereas the *ICD*-11 (2019) provides a more thorough medical perspective, including diagnostic codes for hospitals, Medicare and Medicaid claims, insurance reimbursement, and other health-care-related issues. Even though this could present some confusion, both diagnostic systems emphasize similar criteria.

Cognitive impairment is one of the foremost features of Alzheimer's disease. In order to be diagnosed with major or minor neurocognitive disorder, the patient must demonstrate evidence of a decline from a previous level of cognitive performance. Six cognitive domains may be affected in mild and major neurocognitive disorder, including sustained attention, executive function (e.g., working memory, flexible thinking, and self-control), learning and memory, language, perceptual-motor ability (which allows for skills like hand-eye coordination and object manipulation), and social cognition (such as the ability to identify emotions in others or infer what they might be thinking). Whereas a diagnosis of *major* neurocognitive disorder requires evidence of a *significant* decline affecting at least two domains, diagnosis of *minor* neurocognitive disorder requires *moderate* decline affecting at least one domain. The significance of the person's symptoms is also crucial in determining if cognitive impairment is major or mild. For one to be given a diagnosis of *major* neurocognitive decline, the deficits must be significant enough to evidence a loss of independent functioning (the ability to carry out tasks without the necessary assistance of others, such as feeding oneself, paying bills, or remembering to take medications).

Diagnostic Methods Used to Assess Dementia

A diagnostic approach that involves a physical examination, a clinical interview, a neurological assessment, and neuropsychological testing is often necessary in order to diagnose any form of neurocognitive impairment, including Alzheimer's disease. A physical examination provides information about how certain body systems may contribute to perceived cognitive decline. For example, problems with hearing can affect the ability to follow directions or follow social cues, problems with vision may make it hard to recognize familiar people or objects, and arthritic pain may restrict movement and contribute to disorientation. These factors must be carefully ruled out in order to arrive at an accurate explanation for the cause of a person's subjective report of cognitive decline. A detailed clinical interview is another important part of assessment; it requires patients to describe their major complaints as well as the chronology (a time-ordered progression) of their symptoms. As the patient speaks, a clinician carefully listens and asks clarifying questions in order to uncover further details that may be of clinical importance. External information provided from family members typically offers valuable information at this stage of assessment, because memory decline in patients may make it hard for them to answer important questions about the history of their disease. Neurological assessments, which evaluate the nervous system for motor/sensory deficits, coordination deficits, and motor/sensory problems are especially useful to assess the severity of one's symptoms. One common assessment for neurological decline is the mental-status exam, a semistructured interview protocol that consists of a short series of questions that evaluate a person's behavior, speech, and thought process in order to determine if there are any deficits that may be serious enough to suggest dementia. Another short assessment is the Mini-Mental State Exam, which provides a basic screening for cognitive abnormalities especially compromised by dementia, such as whether a person is oriented to time, place, person, and situation, as well as the person's abilities to utilize short- and long-term memory skills. In some cases of suspected dementia in which a person performs questionably on one of the screening tests, a clinician may make a referral for neuropsychological testing, which involves a battery of different tests that more narrowly assess for specific areas of cognitive difficulty. These tests are not required for a diagnosis of Alzheimer's disease, and they do not help differentiate between one type of dementia or another, but they can be used to more fully identify the cognitive functions that a person may be struggling with, which may, in turn, assist in the treatment planning process. The diagnosis of mild or major neurocognitive decline is usually followed by genotyping tests and/or a neuroimaging assessment in order to find evidence of the suspected origin of the patient's dementia.

Identifying the Presence of Alzheimer's Disease

As described in chapter 1, there are various types of dementia, and each one suggests a different etiology, or cause of disease. Alzheimer's disease is one specific form of dementia that has a unique biological signature in the form of senile amyloid plaques and neurofibrillary tangles—hallmark indicators of the disease first discovered by Alois Alzheimer in 1906 (see chapter 2). In order to qualify for this diagnosis (which is formally termed "major or minor neurocognitive disorder due to Alzheimer's disease"), a person must show *probable* evidence of a genetic or biological indicator (sometimes referred to as a "biomarker" for short) specific to Alzheimer's disease neuropathology. Importantly, the only way to reach a definitive diagnosis of Alzheimer's disease is to conduct a postmortem inspection of brain tissue that successfully reveals the presence of biomarkers unique to Alzheimer's disease (and for this reason, clinical diagnosis of Alzheimer's disease is sometimes rephrased as "probable Alzheimer's disease"). One method to reveal a probable Alzheimer's disease diagnosis is through the use of genotyping, which offers a way of testing for the presence of specific genes that are responsible for coding for specific proteins believed to play a key role in Alzheimer's disease pathophysiology. For instance, the apolipoprotein E (APOE) ε4 variant is typically associated with an increased risk of developing Alzheimer's disease biomarkers. Although genetic tests can provide additional data that may influence an Alzheimer's disease diagnosis, the presence of certain gene variants offers no guarantee that a person will develop Alzheimer's disease (see chapter 8). Neuroimaging is another diagnostic measure that offers a noninvasive way for clinicians to visualize a patient's brain tissue using technologies that inspect the brain for abnormalities in structure or function. For instance, CT (computed tomography) or MRI (magnetic resonance imaging) assessments essentially work by taking pictures of the brain. These methods provide structural imaging of the brain and allow for the detection of shrinkage in key brain areas that may suggest the presence of Alzheimer's disease plaques or tangles. Structural brain imaging also allows the clinician to rule out the possibility of other medical conditions (e.g., cancer) that may explain the patient's reported symptoms. In addition, functional brain imaging utilizes PET (positron emission tomography) or fMRI (functional magnetic resonance imaging) technology that can be ordered to monitor the patient's brain in real time, allowing for the detection of abnormal metabolic processes in certain brain areas that are associated with Alzheimer's disease. However, as the careful reader might anticipate, there is no specific structural or functional neuroimaging finding that allows for a conclusive diagnosis of Alzheimer's disease. Understandably, the diagnostic process can be frustrating for patients, who may feel dissatisfied with diagnostic conclusions that sound ambiguous or speculative. Another aspect that further complicates the diagnosis of Alzheimer's disease is the fact that several completely different diseases can resemble Alzheimer's disease, and each one must first be ruled out before an Alzheimer's diagnosis is made.

Differential Diagnosis

Several psychiatric, neurological, and medical pathologies figure among the diseases that resemble Alzheimer's. For instance, individuals diagnosed with late-life–onset major depressive disorder also experience psychomotor fatigue, reduced movement, and memory impairments.

Depression is known to slow down mental-processing speed and verbal and nonverbal memory, resulting in impaired performance on neuropsychological assessments that measure these aspects of cognition. In fact, episodic memory assessments often fail to properly distinguish patients with Alzheimer's disease from those who have severe levels of major depressive disorder. To complicate matters further, between 30% and 50% of patients with Alzheimer's disease also experience comorbid depression. Clearly, differentiating between the two pathologies is challenging, but it can be done using specialized tests for depression offered by medical or psychiatric professionals.

Even though Alzheimer's disease accounts for the majority of all cases of dementia—60% to 80%, according to the Alzheimer's Association—other forms of neuropathology may better account for a patient's clinical presentation and reported symptoms. For example, vascular cognitive impairment, the second major form of dementia after Alzheimer's disease, accounting for 5% to 10% of cases, is caused by disease that damages the brain's blood vessels. When this happens, blood flow to the brain is restricted, and nerve cells begin to die. Perhaps the best way to distinguish between this condition and Alzheimer's disease is by examining the patient's history of memory loss. If cognitive health seems to decline suddenly and then remain stable after the patient experiences some event that interrupts blood flow (such as stroke), vascular cognitive impairment is the more likely explanation of disease. Lewy body dementia must also be considered as a possible explanation for cognitive decline. This etiology is based on the formation of round, microscopic inclusions that develop inside of brain cells, especially in cell regions that are responsible for memory, thinking, and motor control (movement). While researchers do not know why these abnormal protein deposits form, they do know that their presence is linked to problems with alertness and paying attention but—importantly—not to memory loss. Lewy body dementia can be further distinguished from Alzheimer's disease because of its transient nature: patients experience problems with thinking, but their problems come and go. In addition, patients with Lewy body disease tend to see things that are not real, and this happens regularly in the early stages of disease. In contrast, visual hallucinations are usually seen only at the late stage of Alzheimer's disease. Another dementia, frontotemporal degeneration, refers to a group of genetic disorders that compromise the frontal and temporal lobes of the brain, regions that govern personality, language, and movement. The disease spreads across portions of the frontal and temporal lobes of the brain, and as neurons die, these lobes atrophy (shrink). Frontotemporal degeneration can masquerade as Alzheimer's disease because it also involves a gradual decline in memory, but by contrast, cognitive decline is not one of the first symptoms that patients notice. Instead, dramatic behaviors or personality changes are more likely to be observed first and could include increasingly inappropriate social behaviors, a loss of empathy, and poor judgment. This class of dementias is also known to generate deficits much earlier in a person's life span. Whereas Alzheimer's disease symptoms are most commonly observed after the age of 65, symptoms that indicate frontotemporal lobe degeneration can become apparent as early as age 40. It should also be noted that various medical conditions, such as brain tumors, hydrocephalus, and vitamin B deficiency can also result in cognitive deficits, further underscoring the importance of a careful diagnosis.

CURRENT TREATMENTS

Of course, the deeply concerning nature of Alzheimer's disease warrants questions about the availability of treatment. Although there is no cure for Alzheimer's disease, several pharmacological and nonpharmacological therapies have been developed over the past few decades to assist patients with symptom management and slow the rate of cognitive decline.

Pharmacological Treatments

Drug therapies play an important but limited role in the treatment of Alzheimer's disease. At the time of writing, only five drugs are approved by the U.S. Food and Drug Administration (FDA) for treatment of Alzheimer's pathology, and of these five drugs, none is expected to reverse the disease or halt symptom progression. Medical professionals usually categorize psychotropic drugs based on their mechanism of action, the way that a drug alters brain chemistry to produce a therapeutic effect. All psychotropic medications work by regulating specific neurotransmitters, chemicals that are produced and transmitted between neurons (nerve cells) in the brain. These chemicals affect our thinking, our mood, and our behavior, and when they are not working properly, impairment is observed. Drugs designed to treat Alzheimer's disease typically affect one of two neurotransmitter classes.

Cholinesterase inhibitor drugs work by altering the neurotransmitter acetylcholine (ACh). In the 1980s, it was hypothesized that a depletion of ACh in the brain was the cause of Alzheimer's disease. The nucleus basalis, a part of the brain that seems to be important in attention and memory, is made up of many neurons that are responsible for producing ACh. In Alzheimer's disease, the nucleus basalis is known to deteriorate, and as a result, ACh levels plummet. Importantly, the effect of ACh ends when the neurotransmitter is broken down by a naturally occurring enzyme called acetylcholinesterase (AChE). So, in order to increase the amount of ACh in the brain, cholinesterase inhibitor drugs work by reducing the efficiency of this enzyme so that less ACh is broken down, allowing for more of it to be available in the brain and body. As a result of these higher concentrations of ACh, communication between nerve cells increases and there may be a temporary improvement or stabilization of Alzheimer's symptoms. A 2006 study that involved 13 randomized, double-blind, placebo-controlled trials found that AChE inhibitor drugs such as donepezil (common brand name: Aricept), rivastigmine (Exelon), and galantamine (Razadyne) were shown to be modestly effective in reducing symptoms of mild to moderate Alzheimer's disease. What this means is that people typically score only one or two extra points better on tests of memory and other cognitive functions, however, there is evidence that the drugs can also help improve daily living skills and may improve problematic behavior and emotion patterns. All three drugs were shown to produce similar side effects, unwanted physiological responses that are secondary to the desired therapeutic effect. Common side effects of cholinesterase inhibitors include nausea, abdominal pain, fatigue, headache, vomiting, diarrhea, and insomnia, but these are likely to be reduced as dosages are adjusted each month to better fit the needs of the patient. All three come in pill forms and are taken daily. Rivastigmine is also available in a patch form, which allows for steady absorption and may be a good option for patients who find it difficult to swallow pills or who have stomach problems. However, the patient must remember to change the patch as per physician directions, which may pose a problem for those who suffer from severely compromised memory.

Another popular medication for the cognitive symptoms of Alzheimer's disease is memantine (Namenda), which affects the neurotransmitter glutamate. Glutamate is one of the most common neurotransmitters in the brain and is abundant in the hippocampus, a brain structure primarily involved in memory. Once glutamate is received by a neuron, specific areas of that neuron that are involved in learning and memory, called N-methyl-D-aspartate (NMDA) receptors, become activated. However, NMDA receptors can become overstimulated when there is decreased brain oxygen, which reduces blood flow to the brain. When NMDA receptors are overstimulated by glutamate, calcium rapidly enters the neuron, and it dies because of excitotoxicity (damage due to excessive neurotransmitter stimulation of cell receptors). Memantine functions as a neuroprotective agent that prevents the overstimulation of NMDA receptors by glutamate, allowing neurons to remain healthy. Research suggests that memantine can benefit moderate to severe Alzheimer's patients, and taking 20 milligrams of daily memantine is associated with a 3-point improvement on the 100-point Severe Impairment Battery, a neuropsychological test for severe dementia. Memantine causes no more adverse effects than a placebo does, and side effects are rare, although they include constipation, vomiting, confusion, drowsiness, and hallucinations. The last drug approved by the FDA is also used to treat individuals in the moderate to severe stages of the disease. It is a combination of memantine and donepezil, and its brand name is Namzaric.

Note one important concluding point about medications designed to treat cognitive symptoms: the earlier they are started once symptoms arise, the better. Researchers estimate that the transition from MCI to Alzheimer's disease is as high as 80% over a six-year period. Therefore, early intervention is crucial at the onset of symptoms, as recommended by many studies that have attempted to treat Alzheimer's disease using a pharmacological approach by slowing disease progression. A variety of studies have found that treatment effectiveness tends to be higher in the early stages of Alzheimer's disease than in the later stages.

Several other medications may also be prescribed to assist with emotional or behavioral symptom management for the Alzheimer's disease patient. For instance, when symptoms of aggression, hallucinations, or delusions are reported by caregivers or the patient's family, a class of medications called antipsychotic drugs may be used to reduce such symptoms. Such drugs are typically only prescribed for a duration of less than 12 weeks and are started at extremely low dosages to limit side effects. Physicians also require regular evaluation, usually every 15 days, to ensure the patient's tolerability of antipsychotic medication. Depression in patients with Alzheimer's disease is indicated by appetite problems, disheveled appearance, or crying spells. Antidepressant medications are generally well tolerated by the elderly, but as with all medications, side effects are possible. Caregivers must remain vigilant of any adverse effects that could be attributed to the medication. Because different medication classes carry different side effects, it is best to speak with the prescribing physician to know what to specifically look for.

Nonpharmacological Treatments

Because the pharmacological interventions currently available to treat Alzheimer's disease offer a limited ability to improve symptoms, there has been a growing interest in nonpharmacological treatments that may lead to improvements in a patient's cognition, mood, behavior, and overall quality of life. Such interventions are used not only to improve cognition but also to treat an assortment of behavioral and psychological problems that are often associated with dementia. These may include agitation, restlessness, wandering, disruptive vocalizations, anxiety, resistance to care, depression, delusions, hallucinations, and aggression. According to a 2012 report from the *American Journal of Psychiatry*, 90% of patients with Alzheimer's disease will experience one or more significant behavioral disruptions over the course of their disease. Unfortunately, few medical professionals are instructed about psychosocial interventions or receive information about their effectiveness. As a result, antipsychotic drugs are frequently prescribed before alternative nonpharmacological approaches are even attempted, leading to patients continuing to use possibly risky and unnecessary medications for long periods of time. Concerningly, some research suggests that using antipsychotics to treat dementia offers no better outcome than using a placebo would. In fact, numerous treatment guidelines and specialist groups, such as the American Geriatric Society and the American Association for Geriatric Psychiatry currently identify nonpharmacologic interventions as the preferred first-line treatments for dementia (except for severe cases in which patient behavior is harmful to self or others). Several kinds of nonpharmacological therapies have received empirical attention in recent years. Some of these therapies have been primarily designed to improve aspects of cognition and memory, while others have utilized psychosocial and sensory-based interventions to improve behavioral and emotional functioning.

Cognitive-Based Interventions

Perhaps the nonpharmacologic treatments for Alzheimer's disease that are used most often involve *cognitive training* and *cognitive rehabilitation*, two types of interventions that are used to improve memory and engage thinking. Cognitive-based interventions are believed to work because of neuroplasticity, a quality of the brain that allows it to reorganize its synaptic connections as a result of new experiences. This important brain property makes it possible for the nerve cells to make some remarkable changes in response to guided cognitive stimulation activities. For example, the brain may develop new thinking patterns to compensate for cognitive deficits that compromise memory or attention by recruiting new neural networks to assist with the task, or the brain may modify the strength of its connections between areas responsible for carrying out a certain task (such as hearing, movement, language, or vision). One type of approach, cognitive training, focuses on guided practice to complete tasks that require specific intellectual functions, such as memory, problem-solving, and attention. The major goal of cognitive training is to improve recollection, verbal fluency, attention, comprehension, and executive functions (such as impulse control, self-monitoring, and planning). Cognitive training is often implemented in individual or group settings and may involve different modalities, such as through a computerized touch interface or through more traditional paper-and-pencil formats. The approach is believed to be generally effective. A 2019 Cochrane meta-analysis that reviewed 33 studies and including a total of over 2,000 patients concluded that people who complete cognitive training may experience some benefits in overall cognition, as well as in more specific cognitive abilities such as verbal fluency, and that the results are maintained for at least a few months. However, the report did not find evidence that cognitive training was better than other cognitive treatments such as cognitive rehabilitation or cognitive stimulation.

Cognitive rehabilitation is typically a more complex, individually tailored approach that involves helping patients and their families manage cognitive deficits that are now part of the Alzheimer's patient's reality. Cognitive rehabilitation therapists help patients and their families identify a few specific life areas in which they would like to see improvements. Typically, up to three goals are established, and a therapist assists the patient in developing strategies for achieving such goals. Overall, the focus of cognitive rehabilitation is to improve performance in everyday life functioning rather than to improve scores on specific cognitive assessments. A large-scale trial conducted in 2017 with 475 participants across England and Wales found that cognitive rehabilitation significantly helped people with early-stage dementia improve their ability to gain mastery of deficits that arose as a result of cognitive decline. The goals of patients in this study were varied and were made on a case-by-case basis. For instance, some people wanted to find ways of relearning independence strategies such as using mobile devices or home appliances; others wanted assistance in strengthening their social skills, such as remembering names or improving conversational strategies. Safety was another commonly identified area: patients commonly requested assistance with tasks such as remembering to lock doors or withdrawing money from an ATM. Researchers found that those who participated in the cognitive rehabilitation program, which involved 14 sessions over three months, showed significant improvement in the areas that they identified, and family caregivers agreed that performance improved.

Cognitive training and rehabilitation can be distinguished from two additional cognitive approaches, cognitive stimulation and reality orientation, which offer a group-based approach to rebuilding cognitive abilities for patients experiencing mild and moderate dementia. Essentially, cognitive stimulation operates on the premise that routine cognitive activity builds resistance against the progression of cognitive decline. Patients receiving the treatment become involved with tasks such as discussing current news stories, playing word games together, or doing a practical activity (e.g., cooking) with the support of others. *Reality orientation* is a type of cognitive stimulation aimed at improving the quality of life of confused dementia patients. It involves presenting the patient with continuous personal memory cues (day of birth, occupation, religion, marital status, number of children, children's names) as well as basic temporal and spatial orientation information (such as calendars and information boards that display things such as date, weather, room location, and current events). Patients are encouraged to engage in discussions with group facilitators and other patients on topics such as current news, holidays, birthdays, and other imminent events, and there is strong encouragement for patients to restore social habits and skills they had before the onset of cognitive decline. Although research on the topic is scarce and meta-analytic findings are not available, a 2015 experimental study found positive results: there was significant improvement in the cognitive functioning of Alzheimer's disease patients who completed weekly reality-orientation sessions over a six-month period. Interestingly, the study also found that people who took cholinesterase inhibitor drugs while participating in the reality-orientation program scored significantly higher on a comprehensive neuropsychological battery of tests than did a group who only received pharmacological intervention.

Psychosocial Therapies

In contrast to the cognitive treatments, psychosocial treatments focus more broadly on improving areas of well-being that extend beyond cognition and memory. Although the development of cognitive strategies is an area targeted for improvement, psychosocial treatments put additional emphasis on improving areas such as self-esteem, communication, emotional health, and behavioral management. Reminiscence therapy is one of the most frequently used psychosocial interventions used in treating dementia, and it is particularly known for improving depression. It has been used since the 1980s and is designed to stimulate autobiographical memory. This treatment is typically conducted by a rehabilitation counselor in a group setting, although individually based sessions also exist, which usually involve the guided creation of a life-story book. In either format, the patient is invited to participate in a guided discussion about past activities, events, and experiences. Past familiar belongings, photos, and music are typically used to facilitate memory recollection. The patient's family members are welcomed to participate in the sessions and are commonly involved in the preparation process, which involves choosing which memories are to be targeted for recollection. Research on reminiscence therapy is, unfortunately, limited, but a 2019 study found encouraging results. In the study, reminiscence therapy was provided to 60 late-onset Alzheimer's disease patients, who participated in the treatment sessions for one hour each day over a course of eight weeks. In comparison to a group of Alzheimer's patients who did not participate in the treatment, researchers observed that those who participated in treatment experienced significant treatment gains in terms of reported quality of life, level of depression, and scores on the Mini-Mental State Examination. In addition, a meta-analytic review conducted in 2005 concluded that reminiscence therapy allowed for significant improvements in cognition, quality of life, communication, and mood. These positive effects lasted four to six weeks after treatment.

Validation therapy is another recognized psychosocial treatment that is used in treating dementia at all levels of severity. As its name suggests, validation therapy is based on the general principle of acceptance. All humans have a basic need for approval, reassurance, and connection to others, and those who experience Alzheimer's disease may develop a heightened need for emotional validation as they begin to experience the confusion and distress that follows functional decline. The treatment is centered around the idea that dementia patients can experience a better equality of life if they are able to better communicate their needs and emotions. This is achieved in validation therapy as counselors demonstrate acceptance of their patient's reality and by verbally acknowledging the truth of the patient's experiences. According to Naomi Feil, the social worker who developed validation therapy, its main principles are as follows: (1) All people are valuable, no matter their disorientation; (2) painful feelings that are expressed, acknowledged, and validated by a trusted listener will diminish; and (3) painful feelings that are ignored or suppressed will gain strength. Common parts of a validation therapy session may involve a therapist rephrasing a person's speech back to the person to demonstrate understanding, using factual words to build trust (such as *who, what, when, where,* and *how,* but not *why,* as it could imply judgment), and using a clear, low, loving tone of voice. Unfortunately, research on the effectiveness of validation therapy is limited and contradictory, as the small number of available studies on the topic have drawn different conclusions (this could be due to the difficulty in measuring some of the intended areas of improvement, such as "well-being" or "quality of life"). Meta-analytic studies on validation therapy have found that there is insufficient evidence to conclude that is effective. This does not mean that it is necessarily ineffective—it just means that there weren't strong enough data in past research to suggest that it is clearly helpful. More research will be needed in this area before a better conclusion can be drawn about the usefulness of the treatment.

Sensory Therapies

Sensory therapies, which involve various types of sensory stimulation through light, music, and smell, have also received attention as potential treatments for Alzheimer's disease. Light therapy was initially developed to treat mood disorders and sleep-wake cycle disturbances. It consists of daily light exposure near one's visual field, meant to simulate bright natural light. It has since been used to treat Alzheimer's disease, since 44% of such patients are affected by a sleep disorder. There seems to be a two-way relationship between amyloid plaque buildup and sleep disturbance—in other words, the accumulation of amyloid beta seems to initiate the pathogenesis of Alzheimer's disease, and conversely, the sleep-wake cycle directly influences levels of amyloid beta in the brain. Although many studies have examined the way that light therapy may reduce some of the mood and behavioral problems associated with Alzheimer's disease (such as anxiety, depression, and agitation), only a handful of studies have examined how light therapy can be used to improve cognition. A 2018 meta-analysis that examined the outcomes of five studies on the topic concluded that "all studies have shown modest positive effects on cognition, and one showed that improvements were maintained over time." However, the authors cautioned that the only outcome measure used to evaluate effectiveness was the Mini-Mental State Exam (MMSE), a basic screening test that is not as robust as some of the more advanced neuropsychological tests, which could more thoroughly measure how light therapy affects different aspects of cognition.

Music therapy is defined as the use of music or musical elements (such as sound, voice, or tone) by a qualified music therapist. It is designed to treat cognitive and behavioral effects of Alzheimer's disease by using musical cues to improve autobiographical memory recall. Interestingly, one reason why memories of music may still be retrievable in Alzheimer's disease patients is that the brain regions responsible for music memory do not deteriorate until the later stages of disease, allowing those seemingly forgotten memories to be accessed more easily. In addition, music therapy has been shown to make it easier for dementia patients to encode verbal information either by stimulating or by reducing emotional arousal. In a nutshell, different types of music can affect the autonomic nervous system in different ways by controlling the body's excitement and relaxation responses. These physiological changes have been shown to enhance individuals' ability to maintain attention as they attempt to store newly learned concepts (or experiences) into long-term memory. As a side note, this exact process is the reason behind why the "Mozart effect" is believed to work: listening to classical music does not actually enhance cognition beyond the music-listening session; it only seems to enhance memory because it regulates the nervous system and creates changes in attention quality, which leads to better memory encoding. A 2019 review of music therapy treatments published in the journal *Frontiers in Neuroscience* examined the results of six studies on the topic and concluded that music therapy can positively impact language and memory as well as improve anxiety and depression. However, a few cautions: there is an overall lack of studies on music therapy in general, and many tend to primarily focus on reducing behavioral (not cognitive) symptoms. Only one study found that the benefits of a music therapy program extended beyond the course of a music therapy program. Additional research in this area—such as how music therapy affects the neuropathology of Alzheimer's disease—is still needed.

Stress-Reduction Treatments

Stress is a state of mental or emotional strain or tension resulting from adverse or very demanding circumstances. Stress is especially relevant to Alzheimer's disease in two key ways: it seems to play an exacerbating role in the development of the neurobiological underpinnings of the disease (see chapter 8), and it creates a major source of psychological drain on the lives of those who are diagnosed. Upon learning that one has probable Alzheimer's disease, a sense of alarm, fear, or uneasiness typically sets in as the patient faces distress brought about by changes in lifestyle, autonomy, and identity. Sustained stress levels have also been found to impair episodic memory, a type of long-term memory that allows for the recollection of personal experiences. Elderly individuals living with long-term distress show reduced cognition and an increased likelihood of being diagnosed with cognitive impairment. In addition, higher rates of dementia and worsened cognition are reported in elderly individuals who experience long-term distress.

Stress-reduction programs, especially those that emphasize mindfulness as a method of mitigating distress, have been readily utilized with great success over the past several decades. Mindfulness can be defined as nonjudgmental awareness that arises from training one's attention to remain in the present moment. It is a simple act of paying attention that can be practiced anywhere, at any time, as one becomes especially aware of one's thoughts, feelings, behaviors, and movements. For example, when walking outside on a crisp fall afternoon, we may become especially attentive to the sounds of the wind blowing through the trees, the faint smell of wood burning in the air, and the feeling of warm sunlight on our face. We may also notice that we have anxious or excited thoughts running through our minds, and we may pause for a moment to acknowledge their presence. However, most of us experience life detached from the present moment—our minds wander away from what is happening in the here and now, and we begin to think about things that happened in the past or things that may occur in the future. Mindfulness serves as an anchor that keeps us aware and attentive in the present. In the Buddhist religion, mindfulness serves as one of the practices that lead to the Noble Eightfold Path to enlightenment. Western applications of mindfulness incorporate the technique into secular learning programs designed to reduce distress, over a number of structured sessions.

One of the most popular is mindfulness-based stress reduction (MBSR), an approach that combines a variety of mindfulness techniques with meditation, a more formal, seated practice that serves to calm the mind and create a space where we can intentionally tune into our surroundings and become especially mindful. Over the course of eight weeks, participants learn a variety of mindfulness-meditation techniques that produce reductions in stress, anxiety, hypertension, depression, and neurogenic inflammation—symptoms that each serve as preclinical risk factors that precipitate Alzheimer's disease.

In what has been the largest and most robust study on the topic to date, Spanish researchers conducted a double-blind, randomized, longitudinal study in 2016 to investigate how a new type of MBSR could improve the cognitive skills of patients diagnosed with probable Alzheimer's disease. The study was conducted in Spain and involved 42 participants over the age of 65 who demonstrated significant memory or cognitive impairment. The MBSR program emphasized a variety of components, including attention-to-breathing exercises, a body scan that required patients to pay attention to body sensations (such as heat, cold, and tingling), and some yoga exercises, such as stretching of the arms, legs, head, and torso while using a chair for support, in addition to repeating a verbal mantra while touching the thumb to the other fingers of the hand. The participants also practiced guided mindful attention to body senses, which involved a 10-minute sustained focus on a particular sense, such as smelling incense, visualizing a mountain, touching a smooth surface, or eating a raisin. All treatment sessions took place three days a week for 90 minutes at a time, resulting in an impressive total of 288 sessions over 96 weeks. Researchers examined the cognitive skills of participants before starting the program and again at the end of a two-year period and found that the group demonstrated significantly better scores on a range of cognitive tests. A control group was also monitored over the two-year course of the study and demonstrated no such improvements. Overall, it seems that the long-term practice of stress reduction can be an important preventive measure that could lower the likelihood of cognitive decline among those showing early symptoms of Alzheimer's disease or other related forms of dementia.

Other research studies on meditation have observed treatment outcomes in terms of observed neurological changes within the brain. In 2013, researchers investigated how meditation can improve neuropathology for those with MCI, a transitory state between normal aging and dementia. Fourteen participants completed eight weeks of meditation practice at home each day for an average of 26 minutes. Researchers used functional magnetic resonance imagery (fMRI) at the beginning and end of the study to compare differences in the way that different regions of the brain are connected through neural fibers. After completing the stress-reduction program, the participants showed increased connectivity between the medial prefrontal cortex and the hippocampus—two areas that are specifically affected in Alzheimer's disease. In addition, the participants who completed the stress-reduction training had less hippocampal volume atrophy than control participants. Although this study had a small sample size, it is consistent with other studies that have shown meaningful neural changes after similarly brief meditation interventions. For instance, another eight-week study on a population with MCI found that meditation improved blood flow to the prefrontal cortex—a brain region that is responsible for many cognitive processes that are affected by dementia, such as memory, planning, behavior control, and judgment. Another study found that after only four weeks of meditation training, white-matter neural efficiency increased and improvements in mood were noted, suggesting that meditation may provide faster neurological benefits than was previously believed.

In sum, the host of treatments available for managing Alzheimer's disease are as varied as the assessments that are used to diagnose it. Although we have made significant progress in understanding some of the factors leading to Alzheimer's disease, it is likely that the disease will continue to be a major health problem for some time. Gains in the ability to diagnose the disease and improvements in its treatment offer hope. Over the next several years, treatments based on the known pathogenesis of the disease will become available. Grounded in the significant scientific achievements of the past decade, that is, through 2021, scientists remain hopeful that a cure or preventive treatments will emerge. The next chapter focuses on what patients can expect in the years of their life that follow diagnosis and the initial exploration of treatment options.

6

Long-Term Prognosis and Potential Complications

Prognosis is a clinical word that refers to the predicted course of a disease. It essentially serves as a forecast of what patients and their families can anticipate from a health condition as it is experienced over time. This chapter will focus on the long-term prognosis of Alzheimer's disease, illustrating the types of challenges that can be anticipated after diagnosis. But before examining the progression of Alzheimer's disease and the various complications that can arise from it, we will first need to clear up some misconceptions about what should and should not be expected as a person moves through the later stages of life.

PROGNOSIS AND COURSE OF THE DISEASE

Typical Aging

As mentioned in chapter 1, a myth surrounding aging is the belief that old age will eventually result in cognitive decline. Although it is true that some cognitive deficits occur normally as we age, there is a great misunderstanding of what typical aging actually looks like. Media portrayals of the elderly as excessively forgetful, woefully senile, and dangerously aloof are ubiquitous in movies and television shows. These exaggerated caricatures of the elderly make it easy for us to assume that we are predestined to experience significant cognitive loss as we age. Popular American book titles seem to profit from the public's general fear of aging. A quick search at an online bookstore will yield several titles that reflect our cultural fear of age-related cognitive decline. Zaldy Tan's *Age-Proof Your Mind: Detect, Delay, and Prevent Memory Loss—Before It's Too Late* and Jeff Victoroff's *Saving Your Brain: The Revolutionary Plan to Boost Brain Power, Improve Memory, and Protect Yourself against Aging and Alzheimer's* warn of an inevitable progression from normal aging to alarm-worthy states of distress and disease. This expectation can shape the perceptions people have of elderly family members, neighbors, and strangers, who may be dismissed as "senile" as a result of the misconceptions we have about old age. But in reality, such significant deficits are not the result of typical aging at all. Severe cognitive dysfunction in old age is more often the result of neurological dysfunction (such as dementia or Parkinson's disease), undetected mental illness (such as a mood or anxiety disorder), or medication side effects, which can make some elderly persons appear confused, disoriented, or disheveled. Consider this: old age is always the most common denominator in all of these observations. In other words, old age is easily associated with cognitive decline because we usually see cognitive decline in older individuals and less commonly among younger age groups. This can, unfortunately, lead us to wrongly assume that old age is the *reason* for cognitive decline. Our culturally reinforced expectations, coupled with misattributions made from our own experiences with aging relatives, may lead us to erroneously conclude that severe cognitive deficits are a necessary part of typical aging.

Here's an analogy that further clarifies this crucial point: many Americans experience some type of profoundly stressful experience in their lifetime. It is not surprising that most individuals, even the most mentally healthy ones, will report living through a harrowing experience such as job loss, divorce, or physical trauma. However, most people who experience these psychologically taxing events do *not* subsequently develop major depressive disorder, an abnormal condition often marked by persistent emotional pain, guilt, sleep and eating issues, and, at times, self-harm. Major depressive disorder is not a normal part of development but is more likely among people who have experienced some type of alarmingly stressful life event. The link between aging and Alzheimer's disease is similar. Alzheimer's disease is not the result of normal aging, but it is observed much *more commonly* among elderly individuals than it is among younger individuals. This leads us to incorrectly conclude that old age is *the reason* for symptoms that seem to point to senility, even though the true reason could be due to several other possible causes besides Alzheimer's disease.

The good news is that Alzheimer's disease actually follows a much different course than typical aging, and most older adults will never qualify for any type of dementia diagnosis. In fact, the American Psychological Association reported that fewer than one in five people over the age of 65 (and less than half of those age 85 and older) will ever be diagnosed with any type of dementia. Additional research indicates that even after the age of 85, approximately three-quarters of normally functioning people will not experience significant memory problems. So the question becomes, *What are some of the age-related cognitive problems that are expected as we age normally?* Typical, age-related changes in memory are common and are linked to different brain physiology than what is found in Alzheimer's disease. As we age normally, blood flow to the brain is reduced. The hippocampus, a brain structure responsible for memory storage and retrieval, shrinks and begins to function less efficiently. Levels of brain-derived neurotropic factor (BDNF), a protein used by the hippocampus to repair nerve cells, decline significantly. Although the relationship among these neurophysiological changes is not well understood, their presence is typical of an aging brain. Importantly, age-related cognitive decline is *not* associated with the neurofibrillary tangles and amyloid plaques that characterize the Alzheimer's disease patient's brain (as described in chapter 3), which shows more devastating signs of neurological pathology.

The memory complaints made by people who experience age-related cognitive decline are much less severe than those experienced by dementia patients. For example, a person may report missing a monthly payment, losing things from time to time, or forgetting people's names. Although these experiences may be frustrating, they often do not serve as indicators that one is developing dementia. In fact, these types of memory deficits may seem relatively mild when compared to some of the more dramatic symptoms seen in Alzheimer's disease, such as getting lost in familiar places, losing language skills, and being unable to complete daily living tasks. Normal, age-related cognitive deficits are much less severe and frequent than those observed in Alzheimer's disease.

Fortunately, normal aging does not result in a decline of all types of memory. Cognitive psychologists commonly classify long-term memory into several distinct categories based on the different functions of long-term memory. *Procedural* memory, a type of memory that we use to accomplish performance-based tasks (like playing a musical instrument, riding a bike, or making a cup of coffee) is usually unaffected by normal aging. *Semantic* memory, a type of memory that stores verbal, factual knowledge (such as the name of the state where the Statue of Liberty is located, or the temperature at which water boils) seems to actually *improve* with age, even through one's 70s. Yet other types of memory typically decline with normal aging. Consider *episodic* memory, a type of autobiographical memory that helps us recall aspects of personal experiences—such as where we were and who we were with when the instance occurred. For example, you use episodic memory when recalling your first kiss, where you were on the day of the 9/11 attacks, or what it felt like to ride an airplane for the first time. Sadly, such memories are usually the first type of long-term memory to decline in normal aging and in cognitive decline.

Aside from long-term memory, additional cognitive functions tend to slow down with typical aging, such as the ability to effectively "multitask." Research published in *Proceedings of the National Academy of Sciences* shows that older people, when interrupted, tend to have greater difficulty switching back to their original task than their younger counterparts do. Typical aging also tends to result in measurable decreases in processing speed, an indication of how quickly people can comprehend and reason as they come in contact with new information. This means that as we age, we need more time to interpret and understand numerical information, verbal instructions, and written concepts.

Disease Progression

In the context of Alzheimer's disease, a person's symptoms develop slowly and gradually. Most modern research identifies three general stages of Alzheimer's disease: *early, middle,* and *late* (sometimes referred to as *mild, moderate,* and *severe* in medical contexts). A relatively new clinical period, *preclinical Alzheimer's disease,* is now thought to take place years before a person becomes symptomatic and formally begins to progress through the early, middle, and late stages. Preclinical Alzheimer's disease is therefore understood to be the first phase in the progression of Alzheimer's disease.

There are two important points to keep in mind when examining the course of Alzheimer's disease outlined in this chapter. First, not everyone is expected to follow the same progression. All individuals will experience different symptoms and complications that will shape their unique presentation of the disease. Second, although the course of Alzheimer's disease is presented as a stage model, it often progresses as a continuum. There are blurred boundaries between each stage and no clear indicators that a person has definitively crossed over from one stage to the next. The reason medical professionals tend to think of Alzheimer's disease in terms of various stages is that this type of organization helps patients and their families understand what to generally expect as time goes by, helping them anticipate and prepare for the increasing levels of support that the Alzheimer's patient tends to require.

Preclinical Alzheimer's Disease

The Alzheimer's disease process can begin more than a decade before a person notices any behavioral or cognitive symptoms, as the disease begins to gradually but silently manifest in the affected person's nervous system. The preclinical stage of Alzheimer's disease is typically diagnosed only in research settings, as the affected person usually has no reported need for clinical attention. A preclinical stage is suspected when certain biomarkers that are commonly found in Alzheimer's research become apparent in a patient's brain. Several signs of preclinical Alzheimer's disease have been identified by the Alzheimer's Association Workgroup, and they include detection of the presence of beta-amyloid or tau protein in the nervous system, which can be detected by some newly developed neuroimaging technologies. In addition, if a person's brain shows evidence of gray matter loss or abnormally low metabolic activity in brain regions commonly affected by Alzheimer's disease, a preclinical diagnosis is likely to be given. Because more researchers and physicians are advocating for preventive interventions to be initiated after a preclinical diagnosis is established (see chapter 8), greater attention is currently being placed on this stage and how biomarker assessment can be more regularly integrated into routine medical checkups in the future (see chapter 10). However, it has been observed that most people who develop preclinical Alzheimer's disease will not develop Alzheimer's disease during their lifetimes. In addition, the preclinical period is highly variable in its duration, and for some people, it may extend throughout the life span without ever developing into full-blown Alzheimer's disease. This may create a possible dilemma in the future of dementia assessment, as clinicians and researchers weigh the risk of missing an opportunity for early intervention versus causing distress over what may be a false-positive preclinical indicator.

Mild Alzheimer's Disease: Early Stage

In the early stage, Alzheimer's disease first begins to affect memory, especially short- and medium-term memory. As we age, it is completely normal for us to experience occasional lapses in memory—such as forgetting to pay a credit card bill on time or misplacing car keys. The types of cognitive deficits that Alzheimer's disease patients experience are much more concerning because they occur more frequently and begin to take a toll on multiple aspects of daily life. Although individuals may function independently and remain actively involved in social activities, they begin to notice that they are experiencing difficulties in several important areas. Lapses in long-term memory become a more common occurrence, as they more regularly forget important dates such as birthdays and anniversaries. They may also need a little more time to recognize the face of a longtime friend or family member. Short-term memory becomes less reliable as well, as they find themselves making errors while cooking or remembering to follow through with plans made earlier in the day. They may also need to ask a question multiple times because they have a hard time remembering not only the answer but also the fact that that they already asked the question a short while ago. More recently learned information is less likely to be retained, such as the names of people or places. The ability to perform familiar tasks becomes more effortful, such as following the pattern of a daily routine, planning a family gathering, or remembering the rules of Texas Hold'em. Motor tasks become especially challenging, like typing on a small touch screen keyboard or using tools to perform minor maintenance on a car. Everyday conversation also starts to present challenges for the individual, such as using correct words in conversation (using the word *lake* when the person means to say *pond*). Personality changes may also be observed by family members, as the individual may become more distrustful of others, apathetic, or moody. These deviations are much more likely to affect the individual's relationship with family members, and as such, the person's spouse and children may experience personality changes as more disconcerting than the person's cognitive dysfunctions. All of these symptoms present challenging circumstances for patients and caregivers, but the individual usually does not usually lose the ability to function independently in this stage. Family caretakers may take an increased role in assisting the person with more complex tasks, such as managing finances or facilitating medical appointments, but the person is usually able to perform most essential daily living skills, such as remaining ambulatory, feeding, bathing, and maintaining personal hygiene. However, the individual with mild Alzheimer's disease almost always experiences a progressive worsening of cognitive symptoms while adjusting to a more confusing world in which tasks are more effortful to complete and functioning slows down markedly. However, because many individuals at this stage lack an awareness of their own deficits, they may not see their decline as a cause for concern. They may downplay the severity of their symptoms or insist that they are not experiencing any problems at all. This inability to recognize cognitive deficits will increase with time. In addition, symptoms will continually worsen, and they will continue to experience significant impairments in performing activities of daily living (ADLs).

Moderate Alzheimer's Disease: Middle Stage

As Alzheimer's disease progresses, the individual begins to gradually experience more dramatic symptoms that become more pronounced and difficult to ignore. Moderate Alzheimer's disease is the longest stage, and it can last from 2 to 10 years. As individuals experience greater functional decline in this stage, they may require a greater level of care and assistance. Loss of spatial orientation may appear at this stage as the person becomes more confused about direction and place, resulting in wandering behavior and getting lost in public places. Even familiar settings may become difficult to navigate. Reading and writing, following the plot of a movie, or completing other tasks that involve memory, concentration, and language comprehension present more challenges than ever before. Tasks that require multiple steps to complete, such as doing laundry or making a meal, become especially laborious, due to the requirement that many small actions need to be remembered in sequence and chained together through coordinated muscle movements with good fine-motor execution. Planning and initiating various tasks becomes a challenge, as the individual experiences executive-functioning deficits that make it hard to juggle multiple things at once, like navigating a house while talking on a telephone. Impulse control is another area that falters in the moderate stage of Alzheimer's disease, as a person loses control of potentially inappropriate behaviors, such as interrupting someone who is speaking, saying inappropriate things to others, or touching strangers. Motor skills also decline in this stage, as the individual begins to experience difficulty remaining steady while walking. A cane or wheelchair may become necessary so as to avoid injuries from falling down. The ability to care for oneself independently also begins to decline, as the person may begin to have trouble with tasks that are crucial to daily living, like eating, taking medications, bathing, and using the bathroom. Behavioral and emotional changes, such as restlessness and agitation, also begin to increase in severity. As brain pathology progresses, the person may begin to experience hallucinations (such as seeing shadows, hearing voices, or feeling sensations on the skin that do not exist in reality). The individual may also develop delusional thinking—odd beliefs that are firmly held despite evidence to the contrary—regarding the intentions or behaviors of others. For example, individuals may start to believe that relatives are stealing their money or committing adultery. Increases in agitation also make it all the more difficult for family members to live with the person who is experiencing moderate Alzheimer's disease. Individuals in this stage of Alzheimer's disease can also experience sundowning, a syndrome that occurs in the late afternoon and evening in which a patient experiences considerable confusion or anxiety, displays aggression, or ignores directions. These concerning symptoms will increase until it is no longer appropriate for the individual to live independently. Even if the individual lives with family members, emotional and behavioral symptoms may reach the point that they are too challenging for the family to handle, and caregiving services may be needed to offer additional help in the home environment, at a dementia day care center, or at a permanent assisted living facility.

Severe Alzheimer's Disease: Late Stage

When Alzheimer's disease reaches the final stage, the individual experiences even more debilitating changes that profoundly affect their cognition, daily living skills, and physical well-being. At this stage, neurological damage has spread to the frontal lobe of the brain, which controls several essential processes. In this final stage, nearly all nerve cells of the brain are extensively damaged, aside from the ones that allow for vision and body movement. As a result, cognitive functioning becomes almost completely devastated, and patients will have entered their final stage of life, lasting one to three years. Memory, language, and awareness are reduced to the point of nonexistence as the individual ultimately reaches a point of not recognizing family members, formulating coherent sentences, or even responding to being called by name. Individuals' cognitive functions will become so compromised that they will talk less and less to the point of no longer speaking at all. Daily living skills become similarly reduced. They will experience progressive deficiencies in their movement, beginning with abnormal gait, which will first necessitate a cane and then, when walking is no longer possible, a wheelchair. Individuals will experience additional motor failure in the fingers and eventually in the arms, which will make it difficult to maintain hygiene, put on clothes, and pick up food or a drink. They will also lose the ability to swallow, another motor function that becomes severely reduced in the late stage of Alzheimer's disease. Even when food is put into their mouth, they may forget what to do next. This leads to a high possibility of food getting trapped in the cheeks or the back of the mouth, presenting a heightened risk for choking. For this reason, solid foods may no longer be a safe option for people in the late stage of Alzheimer's disease, and thicker liquids that reduce the risk of choking may be used primarily. In addition to motoric deficits, physical problems appear in abundance at the late stage of Alzheimer's disease. Weight loss is expected to occur as a result of such feeding impairments. Dental problems also become more likely. Because of their nonambulatory status at this stage, individuals are at increased risk for bedsores (injuries to the skin and underlying tissue because of prolonged pressure on bony areas of the body, such as the tailbone, hips, and ankles). The loss of bladder and bowel control will also occur. It will necessitate the use of adult diapers and make the risk of infection from bedsores an important concern, since urine and feces can enter the bloodstream through an open bedsore wound and cause a potentially serious or fatal infection. Urinary tract infections and pneumonia are additional infections that can occur. The loss of such functions will require the individual to be highly dependent on caretakers for basic needs. Because of the extensive needs of individuals at this stage, placement in a nursing home may be needed if the individual is not able to receive sufficient care at home. In cases where the individual experiences terminal medical complications, another option is hospice, which provides comfort and assistance to individuals and families who require end-of-life care.

The stages outlined in this section provide a fairly typical look at how Alzheimer's disease progresses over time. However, as emphasized earlier, all patients' experiences are different in terms of which symptoms are present and which difficulties will arise between diagnosis and the day that the disease ultimately takes their life. It is important for families to learn about the expected course of Alzheimer's disease so that they can know what to anticipate as their loved one progresses through the three stages. The family should be familiar with the symptoms and challenges that are likely to occur throughout this difficult time period. The spouse and children of the patient should have a plan for how they will respond, especially when the patient enters the late stage of Alzheimer's disease and discussions about whether to pursue home assistance, assisted living, or hospice care become necessary. Alzheimer's disease can be a despairing illness, but with knowledge of what to expect, families can significantly reduce their own distress and meaningfully increase the patient's level of comfort.

Disease Prognosis: With versus Without Treatment

It is useful to consider how disease prognosis may differ between people who decide to pursue treatment for their condition (by making lifestyle modifications, taking medication, and/or utilizing nonpharmacological rehabilitation services) and people who do not take such actions. Although some people will want to take advantage of every potentially effective option available, others may question whether it is worth it to take action, because a proactive approach may come packaged with several associated costs. For instance, some patients wonder if accepting medication side effects, financial expenditures, and time commitments will translate to a marked improvement in their day-to-day living experience. The fact that there is no known cure for Alzheimer's disease, coupled with the widespread (but incorrect) belief that nothing can be done to change the outcome of this largely genetic disorder, makes the decision more difficult than it may be in cases of other conditions, such as obesity or diabetes, in which there are stark contrasts between treated and untreated populations in terms of survival rate. Other individuals may never have a choice about whether to begin treatment at all, because they may never receive a correct diagnosis. In fact, according to a 2017 meta-analysis, the proportion of undetected dementia is high—more than 60% of people with dementia are never detected in their communities or in residential nursing care.

Even though it is true that no medication can effectively stop the progression of Alzheimer's disease, there are several outcomes that become more likely if a patient decides to not pursue treatment for symptoms. Perhaps the most obvious difference is a reduction in one's quality of life, as the untreated patient is likely to experience more routine difficulty with completing daily living tasks, like managing money, maintaining personal hygiene, and engaging in tasks that require physical movement if coordination becomes impaired. Faster rates of cognitive decline are also expected if treatment is not pursued, which could lead to losing one's independence earlier in the course of disease. A further problem associated with lack of treatment is increased risk of social isolation. Sometimes, dementia is not diagnosed because people choose to hide their symptoms out of fear of learning what they may mean, and in these cases, they may avoid social contact with friends or family so that the deficits can remain hidden. Receiving treatment for Alzheimer's disease may reduce feelings of loneliness or isolation, as patients may feel more confident in their ability to interact with others.

COMPLICATIONS

In medical terms, the word *complication* refers to any unfavorable outcome that can result from a disease or its treatment. Complications are so named because they "complicate" a patient's experience with a disease. In other words, complications are not directly caused by the disease pathology itself, but they are experienced as secondary consequences that come from having a disease or from receiving treatment for it. For example, Alzheimer's disease is known to produce the symptom of cognitive impairment, which directly results from the brain pathophysiology believed to distinguish Alzheimer's disease from other neurological diseases. Recall from chapter 3 that senile plaques and neurofibrillary tangles are believed to primarily cause cognitive decline. But as a result of memory loss and problems with thinking, a patient may experience the complication of depressed mood. In contrast to disease symptoms, which clinicians carefully assess in order to arrive at a correct diagnosis, complications occur as a secondary process, and they are experienced with greater variation and less predictability. That is why different patients with the same diagnosis can often have very different experiences over the course of their disease.

We have already seen some examples of complications in the "Disease Progression" section earlier in this chapter. That is because complications help characterize and distinguish the different stages of Alzheimer's disease, and they allow patients to anticipate additional challenges that they and their families will likely need to deal with as their condition worsens. It is worthwhile to explore a couple of major categories of complications under a more deliberate focus, because these issues can quickly transform a patient's experience of living with Alzheimer's disease.

Behavioral Disturbances

Behavioral disturbances, a category of complications defined by abnormal changes in behavior, are experienced by nearly all Alzheimer's patients during the course of their disease. Often, these problems can present more difficulties for patients and their caretakers than the more anticipated symptoms of cognitive decline. Because Alzheimer's disease is a progressive neurological disorder that ultimately compromises the function of nearly every area of the brain, it is not surprising that the types of behavioral disturbance observed in Alzheimer's disease are widely varied. We will examine some of the most common behavioral disturbances here.

Depression is a particularly significant behavioral complication that can add an agonizing layer of dysphoria to an already debilitating disease. The Alzheimer's Association estimates that as many as 40% of all Alzheimer's disease patients suffer from clinically significant levels of depression. Clearly, this complication is suspected when a patient reports a decline in mood or seems to develop a fixation on death, but it can also be indicated by some less obvious markers, such as irritability, slowed movement, lack of interest in hygiene, and unexplained aches and pains (which could stem a from psychological origin). Diagnosing depression among this population is challenging, because many Alzheimer's disease patients experience difficulty describing their feelings or reporting how their mood has changed over time, and consequently, the diagnosis is often made based on caregiver observations. A further diagnostic challenge is that there is some overlap between indicators of depression and symptoms known to be caused by Alzheimer's disease itself. For instance, a lack of motivation, sleep disturbance, and decreased appetite may not indicate depression, because these symptoms are known to be manifestations of the pathophysiology underlying Alzheimer's disease. Some research has suggested that the patients at higher levels of risk for developing Alzheimer's disease depression are well-educated, intelligent individuals who often observe their own heartbreaking mental decline. Medication is often used to treat depression, but this can introduce additional complications in the form of side effects, unintended and usually adverse effects that come as a result of taking a drug. Most medications for depression may initially produce side effects, but symptom relief may not follow for up to two months, which is why many antidepressant medications are prematurely discontinued, especially if the side effects are poorly tolerated by the patient. Psychotherapy can also be a viable choice for a patient who seems to experience this challenging complication.

Apathy is a behavioral disturbance that is part of many psychological and neurological disorders, and according to a 2017 review article, it has a mean prevalence of 49%, making it the most common disease complication faced by Alzheimer's disease patients. Apathy can be understood as an absence of motivation, characterized by deficits in behavior (lack of effort or productivity), thought patterns (reduced interest, lack of goals), or emotions (decreased emotional responses). Although this complication frequently accompanies depression, it can also be experienced independently from it. Notably, a few interesting correlations suggest that apathy may serve as an important indicator of disease progression. Apathy not only predicts a patient's current level of functioning but has also been shown to provide a reliable estimate of how long a patient has left to live at any point in time over a 10-year period. Further, patients' level of apathy predicts their overall quality of life, but only if a caregivers' ratings (not patient self-report data) are used. Taken together, this suggests that apathy may be understood as a serious complication that could be used to improve the accuracy of a patient's current prognosis and that caregivers should be especially vigilant for its signs. Although medication is unlikely to treat apathy, a recent review on nonpharmacological treatment of apathy in Alzheimer's disease concluded that some improvements might be possible with one-on-one activities, kit-based activity interventions, cognitive rehabilitation, and other individualized therapy programs.

Wandering is another expected complication that can create challenges for Alzheimer's disease patients and their caregivers. Wandering is observed when a patient walks almost aimlessly, often getting inside of things such as closets and attics. Although the in-home wandering of some patients is mostly harmless, the seriousness of the behavior magnifies if a patient is prone to falling down or making frequent attempts to leave a residence without others noticing. This is an area of concern because the consequences of wandering and getting lost outside the home can range from minor injuries to death, and if a person is not found within 24 hours, there is up to a 50% chance that the person will die or sustain a serious injury. According to a 2018, literature review, more than 60% of people who live at home will wander, but the statistic drops to 23% if people live in a nursing home. Therefore, if Alzheimer's disease patients begin to demonstrate wandering behavior that jeopardizes their safety, it may be important for caregivers to consider the possibility of pursuing assisted living arrangements or hiring a caretaker to provide more routine supervision. However, doing so may require the patient's family to incur a significant financial burden. Wandering used to be treated with the use of physical restraints and medications, but today, different approaches that allow the patient to retain some degree of autonomy are preferred. These include high-tech solutions, such as GPS tracking devices as well as simple ones, such as using mirrors to disguise doors, placing distractions near barriers, or engaging patients in exercise programs.

Aggression and agitation can significantly complicate a patient's prognosis. People who have been diagnosed with Alzheimer's disease or mild cognitive impairment (MCI) are five times more likely to develop aggression, which could manifest in a verbal form (shouting, using profane language, hurling verbal insults) or through some kind of physical action (hitting, throwing objects, biting). In almost all cases in which aggression is reported, it creates serious daily stress for the patient and the caregiver. A 2019 meta-analysis published in the *American Journal of Geriatric Psychiatry* reported that aggressive behaviors "are among the most frequent and disruptive behavioral complications of cognitive decline" and that they are one of the major contributors to increased costs of living, hospitalization, and premature institutionalization, as well as caregiver depression. Aggression can develop due to a variety of reasons, but one common reason is physical discomfort. According to the Alzheimer's Association, the patient may experience physical discomfort as a result of medication side effects, feeling hungry or thirsty, or inadequate sleep. Environmental factors are another main cause of aggressive behaviors. Loud noises, unfamiliar people, and large crowds can be overwhelming for an Alzheimer's disease patient and can cause considerable distress. Communication problems may also lead to aggressive reactions, as a patient may become frustrated when caretakers ask confusing questions or when they ask multiple questions before the patient has time to respond. Notably, a source of frustration can come from the fact that patients may experience communication problems themselves, that is, when they cannot articulate their own discomfort. Patience, redirection tasks, taking breaks, and a good amount of empathy are often needed to reduce aggressive behavior, but when the problem is unabating or if it becomes more severe, medication may be prescribed.

Medical Complications

Although Alzheimer's disease is most easily recognized as a disorder involving memory and cognition, several medical complications can result from it that could present significant health risks to the patient. Although it is beyond the scope of this book to identify all of the physiological issues that could develop between the time of diagnosis and death, a few medical complications are worth mentioning because of their widespread prevalence. Aphasia, or loss of speech and language comprehension abilities, affects many Alzheimer's patients. It usually begins with a loss of reading comprehension, and as the disease progresses, patients may begin to stumble over their words or they may start to speak using a random mixture of words and phrases that do not make sense. There is some evidence that Alzheimer's disease medication, especially Memantine and Donepezil, can slow the progression of aphasia. Gait disturbances, or problems with walking, are another regularly expected outcome of Alzheimer's disease, especially in the middle and late stages. This issue could manifest as unsteadiness while walking, making it more likely that the patient will lose balance and fall. For this reason, physical therapy sometimes becomes part of the treatment regimen, which can correct some gait issues through leg stretching and strength-building exercises. A mobility device, such as a walker or a cane, will also be necessary for most patients who experience gait problems. Incontinence can further complicate a patient's experience with Alzheimer's disease in the later stages. This problem can occur when mobility issues prevent a patient from getting to a toilet on time. Or it could be due to a decline in language skills, which may make it difficult for patients to alert caregivers that they need to use a restroom. It is also possible that a patient may forget how to use a toilet or where one is located, further contributing to accidents. Weight loss and eating problems are other common complications that occur in the later stages, as patients regularly lose the ability to feed themselves and, ultimately, their ability to chew and swallow. Difficulties ingesting food can be extremely worrisome—not only can they cause choking but they often result in a dangerous lung condition called aspiration pneumonia. This kind of infection occurs when improperly swallowed food gets lodged inside the lungs, and it is the most common cause of death among people with Alzheimer's disease. To protect against it, caregivers will need to ensure that ample time is given for eating (often up to 60 minutes) and that the patient's diet is made up of liquids and soft, easy-to-swallow foods.

Overall, the course of Alzheimer's disease is highly variable and largely unpredictable. Although most patients will experience the same gradual decline in cognitive and physical health, a unique pattern of distressing symptoms and difficult complications are often part of every patient's experience with the disease. The challenging effects of Alzheimer's disease often extend beyond the patient as well. The next chapter focuses on the demands placed on family members and caregivers, who often face significant pressure of their own in dealing with the outcomes of the disease.

7

Effects on Family and Friends

According to the Alzheimer's Association, caregiving refers to attending to another person's health needs and well-being. In the United States, family members, relatives, and other unpaid caregivers provide more than 80% of the assistance to older adults. Almost half of all caregivers who assist older adults do so with someone who has Alzheimer's disease or another type of dementia. Caring for someone who has Alzheimer's disease can be physically, emotionally, and financially draining. The demands of everyday care, changes in family roles, and decisions about whether your loved one should be at home or in a care facility can be difficult. This chapter focuses on the impact Alzheimer's has on the family and friends of the individual living with the disease.

WHO ARE THE CAREGIVERS?

The demographic background of those caring for individuals with Alzheimer's or other dementias varies. However, several sources including the U.S. Department of Health and Human Services, the National Alliance of Caregiving, and the Alzheimer's Association reveal some common characteristics of these caregivers. The majority of caregivers live with the person with dementia, and the majority are women. Over half of caregivers are providing assistance to a parent or in-law with dementia. Of those caring for an aging parent or in-law, many have children of their own they need to care for as well. Approximately 10% of caregivers provide help to a spouse with Alzheimer's disease or another dementia. In addition, about one-third of caregivers are older adults (i.e., those age 65 or older). Non-Hispanic white caregivers make up two-thirds of the workforce, while Black/African American caregivers make up 10%, Hispanic/Latino caregivers make up 8%, and Asian caregivers make up 5%. The rest are from various racial and ethnic backgrounds. Around 40% of caregivers have a bachelor's degree or further education. A household income of $50,000 or less is the standard for 41% of caregivers.

WHAT TO DO WHEN YOU NOTICE A CHANGE IN A LOVED ONE

Recall from chapter 4 that memory loss that interferes with everyday life, difficulty organizing or solving problems, difficulty performing familiar tasks, confusion with time or location, problems speaking or writing, misplacing items and losing the ability to retrace one's steps, impaired judgment, sudden detachment from activities, and changes in mood or personality are all common warning signs of Alzheimer's disease. If you notice these changes in friends, family, or others close to you, and you are concerned, it can be difficult to know what to do or say. Although it is typical to be uncertain or worried about how to offer support, these are considerable health concerns. The Alzheimer's Association provides helpful suggestions to take action. The first thing to do is to assess the situation. Think about what changes in memory, thinking, or behavior have occurred. In addition, assess whether something else may be occurring that could be responsible for these changes. For example, is the person taking a new medication, or has the person experienced a recent stress in life such as the loss of a job or loved one? One or more of these may play a role in the changes you are seeing. Also, find out if anyone else has noticed these changes as well. Next, take action through communication. You should have a conversation with your loved one along with another family member or friend about your concerns. Do not wait to have the conversation; instead, have it as soon as possible. The earlier the individual gets help, the better the prognosis. When having the conversation, choose a date, time of day, and place where the individual feels most comfortable. You may have difficulty knowing what to say, so make sure you let them know your concern. You might start by saying, "How have you been feeling lately?" or "I noticed you [give a specific example] and it worried me. Has anything else similar to that happened?" Also, it is best for you and one other person to be present rather than a large group of people so that your loved one does not feel threatened or ambushed. If the first conversation is not successful, have more than one conversation. Sometimes it takes more than one conversation for the individual to seek help. Lastly, offer to go to the doctor with the person. This shows you are supportive of the person finding out what is causing the problems. And it is always good to have a second person present when speaking with a physician in order to write down what was said and advised as to next step(s).

PAID VERSUS UNPAID CAREGIVERS

Individuals who care for those with Alzheimer's are called direct-care workers. Their job is to give assistance to the elderly, individuals with a physical or intellectual disability, or those who are sick or injured. According to the U.S. Bureau of Labor Statistics, direct-care workers fall into three main categories: nursing assistants, home health aides, and personal care aides. Nursing assistants generally work in nursing homes, although some work in assisted living facilities, other community-based settings, or hospitals. Nursing assistants make up the bulk of the staff in nursing homes who deal with cognitively impaired residents. The majority of nursing assistants are female, and they come from a variety of ethnic, racial, and environmental backgrounds. They assist residents with activities of daily living (ADLs), such as food preparation and eating, dressing, bathing, and going to the bathroom. They also perform some medical activities, such as range-of-motion exercises and blood pressure readings. Home health aides have virtually the same roles as nursing assistants but are under the direction of a nurse or therapist; they support people in their homes or in community settings. They may also be responsible for light housekeeping duties, such as changing linens, meal planning, and administering prescriptions in addition to ADL assistance. Additionally, they may help people get to work and become involved in their communities.

Direct-care staff have tough careers, and they may not be well trained to care for people with dementia. Turnover rates are high, and recruitment and retention are constant challenges. Inadequate education and challenging work environments have also contributed to higher turnover rates among nursing staff across care environments. Only nursing assistants and home health aides who work in Medicare- and Medicaid-certified nursing homes and home health agencies are required to complete training. Other types of direct-care staff, on the other hand, may be required to complete training or certification by states or individual employers.

Professionals who may receive special training in caring for older adults are physicians, nurse practitioners, registered nurses, social workers, pharmacists, physician assistants and caseworkers. According to the American Association of Nurse Practitioners, there are over 290,000 licensed nurse practitioners currently in the United States. However, just under 8% of nurse practitioners are certified in adult gerontology primary care. Furthermore, only about 1% of registered nurses, physician assistants, and pharmacists describe themselves as geriatrics specialists. Despite the fact that 73% of social workers work with people ages 55 and up, only 4% of them are certified in geriatric social work. In addition, the number of paid caregivers could be affected by the overall aging of the long-term-care workforce. According to the Eldercare Workforce Alliance, as the number of older adults increase, it is estimated that by 2030, 3.5 million additional health-care professionals and direct-care workers will be needed.

Paid workers are not the only people who care for individuals with Alzheimer's disease and other dementias. In fact, the majority of people caring for these individuals are unpaid workers. More than 16 million Americans provide unpaid care for people with Alzheimer's or other dementias. According to a 2017 study published in the *Journal of the American Geriatrics Society*, 70% of the lifetime cost of care is shouldered by family caregivers in the forms of unpaid caregiving and out-of-pocket expenses for necessary items such as medication or food for the person with dementia. In 2019, caregivers of people with Alzheimer's or other dementias provided over 18 billion hours of unpaid assistance. In 2019, the total lifetime cost of care for someone with dementia was estimated to be over $350,000. This is very costly for individuals. Recall that just over 40% of caregivers have a household income of $50,000 or less. So why would someone be an unpaid caregiver?

According to the Alzheimer's Association, there are three main reasons caregivers provide care and assistance to a person with Alzheimer's or other dementia: (1) they want to keep the family member or friend at home, (2) they want to be in close proximity to the person, or (3) they feel obligated to take care of the person. A 2019 review of the literature regarding people's motivations for being unpaid caregivers revealed that people's motives were frequently based on their relationship with the person and on emotions such as love and wanting to reciprocate care received from the person in the past. Caring for the family member has not usually been regarded as something extraordinary but rather as a typical part of family life. It has often been described as an obligation or responsibility. The researchers also found that caregiving was rarely driven by one motivation alone; rather, people often had multiple motivations for caring for a loved one living with Alzheimer's or other dementia. Just a small number of dementia patients do not receive assistance from relatives or other informal caregivers. Nearly half of these people live alone and find it more difficult to ask for and obtain help. For certain people, living alone with dementia may be very difficult. Lesbian, gay, bisexual, and transgender (LGBT) people, for example, may feel more isolated as a result of social stigma or a smaller social network of available family or friend caregivers.

CAREGIVERS' TASKS

The care provided to people with Alzheimer's or other dementias is wide ranging. Caregivers help with instrumental activities of daily living (IADLs), such as household chores, shopping, preparing meals, providing transportation, arranging for medical appointments, and managing finances. They help the person take medications correctly as well as make certain they stick to treatment recommendations for dementia or other medical conditions. In addition, caregivers assist with personal ADLs, such as bathing, dressing, grooming, feeding, helping the person walk, and changing the person's position—for instance, moving the person from bed to chair. As discussed in chapter 4, individuals with Alzheimer's may experience mood and/or personality changes. Therefore, caregivers often need to manage behavioral symptoms of the disease, such as aggressive behavior, wandering, depressive mood, agitation, anxiety, repetitive activity, and sleep disturbances. In addition to providing assistance with various ADLs, caregivers may also need to find support services; make arrangements for paid in-home care, nursing home, or assisted living care; or hire and supervise others who provide care. When a person with Alzheimer's disease or another form of dementia transitions to an assisted living facility or a nursing home, the assistance offered by the caregiver of the family typically shifts from comprehensive treatment to emotional support, communicating with facility staff, and advocating for proper care. However, some family caregivers continue to help with some ADLs.

Not all tasks involve ADLs. Caregivers may assume additional responsibilities that are not necessarily specific tasks. For example, they may be responsible for day-to-day management or family problems related to caring for a relative with Alzheimer's disease, such as contact with other family members about care plans, decision-making, and respite care arrangements.

Though family members of people with Alzheimer's or other dementias provide treatment that is comparable to that given by caregivers with people with other conditions, dementia caregivers appear to provide more comprehensive assistance. Caregivers of people living with dementia are more likely than caregivers of people without dementia to track the health of the care recipient. Caregivers of people living with dementia are more likely than caregivers of people without dementia to provide assistance with self-care, mobility, and medical care, according to data from the 2011 *National Health and Aging Trends Study.*

CAREGIVER HEALTH AND WELL-BEING

The demands of caregiving can cause some caregivers' health to deteriorate. The burden of delivering care to those living with dementia has been shown to raise caregivers' vulnerability to illness and other health complications. Caregiving-related chronic stress has been linked to an increased occurrence of high blood pressure and a variety of physiological changes that may increase the risk of developing chronic conditions, such as elevated stress hormone levels, weakened immune function, and coronary heart disease. According to the Alzheimer's Association, 38% of Alzheimer's and other dementia caregivers indicate that the physical stress of caregiving is high to very high. Based on these findings, it should be no surprise that a 2018 study published in the journal *Neurological Sciences* found that as the disease progresses, the burden on caregivers increases and their mental health begins to decline. In that same year, a review of the literature regarding the mental health of caregivers (as opposed to non-caregivers) found that caregivers of people with dementia were significantly more likely to experience depression and anxiety than non-caregivers were. Caregivers of individuals living with Alzheimer's indicate more cognitive issues, such as memory difficulties, and experience more cognitive loss over time than non-caregivers do. In addition, there seems to be a threshold for caregivers' mental health regarding the number of behavioral and psychological symptoms the person living with Alzheimer's exhibits. Paul Arthur and colleagues found that caring for dementia patients with four or more behavioral and psychological symptoms, such as agitation, self-harm, trouble writing, and wandering, is a "tipping point" for family members, as they are more likely to experience depression and negative emotional reactions to providing care.

According to a 2017 *National Poll on Healthy Aging,* nearly three-fourths of caregivers of people with Alzheimer's or other dementias reported that they were "somewhat concerned" to "very concerned" about maintaining their own health since becoming a caregiver. Furthermore, 27% of dementia caregivers postponed or failed to do something that they should have done to protect their own well-being. Dementia caregivers have a poorer health-related quality of life than non-caregivers and are more likely to say their health is fair or poor than non-caregivers. Given these numbers regarding their own health, it should be no surprise that 35% of caregivers of people living with Alzheimer's or another dementia claim their health has deteriorated as a result of their caregiving duties, compared to 19% of caregivers of people without dementia.

Because of the memory loss, functional disability, and behavioral disturbances that may accompany the development of Alzheimer's disease, the trust, shared interactions, and memories that are often part of the partnership between a caregiver and an individual living with dementia can be at risk. However, a 2010 study in the journal *Psychology and Aging*, the effects of helping depend on the nature of the relationship between the caregiver and the recipient of care. Helping produces positive rather than negative emotions in caregivers who see themselves as highly interdependent (sharing a common fate) with the person. Caregivers' well-being may be enhanced by assisting loved ones. Furthermore, the 2017 *National Poll on Healthy Aging* showed that 45% of caregivers of people with dementia indicated that providing help to someone with cognitive impairment was very rewarding. It is worth noting that, while caregivers often express positive feelings about their work, such as family togetherness and the satisfaction of helping others, they also often express high levels of stress. The burden of caring for a loved one with Alzheimer's or another dementia has been shown to have a negative impact on the sleep quality of family caregivers. According to a 2019 review of caregivers' sleep duration and quality, caregivers of people with dementia lose between 2.4 and 3.5 hours of sleep per week relative to those of the same age who are not caregivers.

As a caregiver, delaying or not maintaining one's own health is not beneficial to anyone. You can find that you have so many obligations that you forget to look after yourself. However, staying physically and emotionally strong is the best thing you can do for the person you are caring for. The following are some suggestions from the National Institute on Aging (NIA) of ways to take care of yourself. First, ask for help when you need it. Trying to do everything by yourself will leave you exhausted. Seek support from family, friends, your faith community, or a caregiver's support group. Second, take breaks every day. It is typical to need a break from caregiving duties; no one can do it all by themselves. Third, keep up with your hobbies and interests. Spending time doing something you enjoy can help your overall mental health and well-being. People who participate in hobbies are less likely to experience stress, a depressed mood, or depression. Fourth, eat healthy. Healthy eating, such as the DASH (Dietary Approaches to Stop Hypertension), Mediterranean, or ketogenic diets, are good for overall health and may help protect the brain. DASH and Mediterranean diets emphasize whole grains, fruits, vegetables, fish, nuts, and olive oil and other healthy fats; a ketogenic diet limits the amount of carbohydrates a person takes in. Chapter 8 discusses in greater detail dietary factors associated with reducing one's risk of Alzheimer's. Fifth, be active. Everyone knows that exercise is an important part of staying healthy. It has been shown to help relieve stress, prevent disease, and make you feel good. But finding the time to exercise can be difficult. Here are some helpful tips to incorporate exercise into your routine:

- Start small. While getting 30 minutes of physical activity at least five days a week is recommended, you can benefit from even 10 minutes a day.
- Accept offers of assistance from friends and family. In a short amount of time, you can get in a good workout.
- Take advantage of exercising when the person with dementia takes a nap. You can pull out a mat to stretch, ride a stationary bike, or simply walk up and down the stairs several times.
- Find something you enjoy. It will be easier to form a habit if you like the activity. Also, depending on the severity of the disease, you can incorporate exercise into your loved one's routine as well. For example, you can take a walk together, participate in exercise videos, dance together to favorite music, throw a soft ball or balloon back and forth, garden, or do other activities you both enjoy.
- Regularly visit your physician and listen to your body. Ignoring symptoms such as exhaustion, sleeplessness, or changes in appetite can cause your physical and mental health to decline.

To cope with the issues of caregiving and help maintain your overall health and well-being, keep a few things in mind. Remember that the treatment you provide matters and that you are doing your best. You may feel guilty because you cannot do more over time, but do not forget that care needs will change as the disease progresses. People living with Alzheimer's change over time and so do their needs; accept changes as they occur. Grieve the losses, but more importantly focus on positive times as they arise, and enjoy good memories. Be mindful that your loved one may need treatment beyond what you can offer on your own at some point. You can make the transition easier by learning about community resources and care options, such as home care or residential care.

CAREGIVER STRESS

Taking care of anyone can be stressful, however caring for someone living with Alzheimer's or another dementia can be especially stressful. As we learned in chapter 5, stress is a state of mental or emotional strain brought on by difficult or challenging circumstances. It seems in this day and age that everyone is stressed. But how do we know if we are experiencing stress because we are taking care of someone? The Alzheimer's

Association presents various symptoms of caregiver stress: denial, anger, anxiety, depression, irritability, lack of concentration, exhaustion, social withdrawal, sleeplessness, and health problems. You may find yourself in denial about the disease or the effects it has on your loved one. You may be angry at the person living with Alzheimer's or frustrated that the person can no longer do the things the person was once able to do. You may be anxious or depressed because you do not know what the future holds. You may find that the smallest things set you off or you have no patience for anything. Since you are so busy, you may have trouble remembering things or you may be exhausted, which makes it nearly impossible to complete everything that is needed to be done that day. You may find yourself withdrawing from friends and activities that used to be a source of enjoyment for you. You may have trouble sleeping, caused by a never-ending list of concerns such as worrying about the person falling out of bed or wandering off in the middle of the night. You may experience health problems that begin to take a mental and physical toll on you; you may not remember the last time you felt good. Make an appointment with your doctor if you notice any of these symptoms of stress on a regular basis. As mentioned in the section above on caregiver health and well-being, it is important for you to maintain your health just as much as the health and well-being of the person you are taking care of.

We know that stress can trigger physical problems, such as blurred vision, stomach pain, or high blood pressure, as well as behavioral changes such as irritability, loss of focus, and appetite changes. Therefore, it is important, not only for you but also for the person you are caring for, that you find effective ways to manage your stress. Recent research in the *Journal of the American Geriatrics Society* has emerged on the effects of caregiver stress on people with dementia and their use of health-care services. For instance, Nathan Stall and colleagues found that distress on the part of family caregivers is associated with the increased likelihood of the person with dementia being institutionalized, worsened behavioral and psychological challenges in the person with dementia, and the increased likelihood of people with dementia being abused. The demands of caregiving may intensify as people with dementia approach the end of life. A study titled the "End-of-Life Care and the Effects of Bereavement on Family Caregivers of Persons with Dementia" found that 59% of caregivers felt they were "on duty" 24 hours a day in the year leading up to the death of the individual living with dementia, and many felt caregiving was particularly stressful. Additionally, when the person with Alzheimer's or another dementia passed away, 72% of family caregivers felt relieved.

The Alzheimer's Association has tips for caregivers to help manage their stress. Some of these are similar to the suggestions from the NIA on ways to take care of yourself, as discussed in the previous section:

- Get help when needed, and find support by knowing what resources are available. Adult day programs, in-home support, visiting nurses, and food delivery are only a few of the resources available to assist you with ADL (activities for daily living) management. There are many resources listed in this book's "Directory of Resources" that you may find helpful. One resource in particular is the Alzheimer's Navigator from the Alzheimer's Association. It creates a customized action plan for caregivers and connects them to information, support, and local resources.

- Make use of relaxation methods. There are a number of basic relaxation methods that can aid in stress relief. Some examples of relaxation methods are visualization, meditation, breathing exercises, and muscle relaxation.

- Engage in any form of physical activity. As discussed, exercise can help reduce stress and improve overall well-being.

- Find some time for yourself. If you do not want or are not able to ask another family member or friend, professional respite care can provide a temporary break from caregiving, while the person with Alzheimer's continues to receive care in a safe environment. Examples of respite care are in-home care services, adult day centers, and residential facilities. Using respite services can reduce your stress and strengthen your ability as a caregiver.

- Take care of your health. Regularly see the doctor, eat well, and get plenty of rest. Maintaining your well-being will assist you in being a better caregiver.

- Become a well-informed caregiver. New caregiving skills may be required as the disease progresses. There are several services available to assist you with better understanding and coping with the behaviors and personality changes that often accompany Alzheimer's disease. Talking to other caregivers about how they are dealing with the disease's challenges and anxiety about the future can also be beneficial.

- Make legal and financial preparations. Following an Alzheimer's diagnosis, it is critical to put legal and financial arrangements in place so that the individual living with the disease can participate. Having future plans in place will give the entire family peace of mind. Without the assistance of an attorney, several records may be prepared. If you're uncertain how to fill out legal paperwork or make financial arrangements, you may want to seek help from an elder law attorney, a financial planner who is familiar with elder or long-term-care planning, or both.

FINANCES

In addition to the changes that occur over the course of Alzheimer's disease, many families will experience a significant financial burden as a result of the high costs associated with caregiving and treatment. The total direct cost of care for the treatment of Alzheimer's disease in 2020 was estimated to be $305 billion, according to the *American Journal of Managed Care*. Total Medicare costs in 2019 were estimated to be $25,213 (per person) for people living with Alzheimer's disease or other forms of dementia. That figure is more than three times higher than the Medicare expenditures for people who do not experience a form of dementia. Medicaid covers the costs of long-term-care services for patients with low income who meet certain eligibility criteria. The average 2019 Medicaid payment toward services needed for a patient with Alzheimer's disease was a whopping $8,779—more than 23 times higher than the cost paid by Medicaid to individuals with other conditions ($374). Moreover, the average annual per-capita out-of-pocket spending was estimated at $3,285, which is 57% higher than out-of-pocket spending of patients who did not have the disease or a related dementia ($1,895). It is clear that Alzheimer's disease causes significant economic and financial strain.

A less apparent but perhaps more significant strain is associated with the indirect costs of the disease, such as loss or reduction of income by family members who become caretakers. As mentioned earlier in this chapter, out of obligation and love, and through an effort to keep a loved one comfortable in their own home during a difficult period of life, family or friends often take on the burden of providing unpaid care to an Alzheimer's disease patient who shows signs of needing routine assistance. This type of care is believed to make up over 80% of all caregiving for Alzheimer's disease patients, according to an estimate by the *Journal of the American Geriatric Society*. That is a staggering figure, especially when it is further understood that the act of providing caregiving services to a loved one with Alzheimer's disease is no small task—the disease course is characteristically longer in duration than other disorders, and it causes unrelenting physical and cognitive declines in functioning. Many informal caretakers not only assist their loved one with daily life activities (e.g., getting dressed, eating, retrieving the mail), but they also play a key role in managing other challenging or time-consuming tasks such as ensuring medication compliance, helping a patient cope with behavioral disturbances of the disease, or making arrangements for supportive services (such as adult day programs, medical appointments, or forms of in-home care). As the patient's overall level of functioning declines, family caregivers may need to reduce their working hours to care for the patient, which often translates to lost wages as caregiving evolves into an increasingly time consuming and costly responsibility. In addition, data from the Alzheimer's Association Family Impact of Alzheimer's survey revealed that caregivers often cut back on spending and on saving due to the out-of-pocket costs of providing help to someone with dementia. An intriguing study, published in 2018 by the *Journal of the American Geriatric Society*, estimated the total costs incurred by informal caretakers over a two-year period. When basing the estimate from lost wages alone, it was estimated that the median cost of informal caretaking was $24,000. But when a more robust prediction was made that accounted for other indirect monetized costs to the caretaker, such as lost leisure time, reduced future employability, and expenditures for health and well-being, the median cost of informal caregiving was much higher—$180,000 over two years—about the same cost as full-time residential care. This finding suggests that the financial burden associated with informal caregiving is often greater than what may be expected from predictions based on lost wages alone.

SUPPORT FOR CAREGIVERS

For more than three decades, strategies or interventions to support family caregivers of people with Alzheimer's and other dementias have been developed and evaluated. The aim of these measures is to strengthen dementia caregivers' health and well-being by reducing the negative aspects of caregiving. Some programs also seek to delay the individual with dementia's transition to a care facility by equipping caregivers with the expertise and resources they need to continue supporting their loved ones at home. Case management, psychoeducational methods, counseling, psychotherapeutic approaches, education, assisting caregivers in managing dementia-related symptoms, strengthening social support for caregivers, and providing caregivers with respite from caregiving duties are some of the specific approaches utilized in different intervention strategies. According to the Alzheimer's Association, case management provides assessment, information, planning, referral, and care coordination for caregivers. Programs that offer knowledge about the disease, resources, and services, as well as about how to improve skills to effectively react to disease symptoms, are examples of psychoeducational approaches. Counseling helps address preexisting personal issues that hinder caregiving, mitigate conflicts between caregiver and care recipient, and/or improve family functioning. The development of a therapeutic partnership between the caregiver and a mental health provider is central to psychotherapeutic approaches. Psychoeducational and psychotherapeutic interventions are more formal than support groups. They enable caregivers to express personal feelings and concerns, which can help alleviate feelings of isolation. As mentioned previously, respite care comes in various forms, such as in-home care services, adult day centers, and residential facilities, to provide temporary relief for the caregiver. A 2017 study focusing on the effectiveness that mindfulness has as an intervention for caregivers found that mindfulness interventions showed significant effects of improvement in depression, perceived stress, and mental-health-related quality of life at two months after treatment.

According to a 2015 publication on dementia caregiver interventions in *The Gerontologist*, successful interventions actively included family caregivers in the intervention. When an intervention is personalized and adaptive to meet the changing needs of family caregivers over the course of the disease, it is also successful. Finally, the intervention should address the needs not only of caregivers but also of those living with dementia. More recent research published in *The Gerontologist* looked at the most effective elements of dementia caregiver treatments. The researchers discovered that strategies that first enhance competency ability of caregivers, then gradually address the care needs of the individual living with dementia, and finally provide emotional support for loss and grief when needed tend to be the most successful.

There is some indication that families are now better at managing the care they provide to relatives with dementia than in the past. A longitudinal study from 1999 to 2015 found that dementia caregivers were significantly less likely to report physical difficulties related to providing care. In addition, use of respite care by caregivers of individuals living with a dementia increased over time. However, more work is needed to ensure that interventions for dementia caregivers are available and accessible to those who need them. For instance, a 2016 report of the National Family Caregiver Support Program found that over half of Area Agencies on Aging did not offer evidence-based family caregiver interventions.

This chapter has focused on the ways Alzheimer's impacts family and friends of those living with the disease. Becoming well informed about the disease is an important aspect for caregivers of individuals with Alzheimer's or other dementias. Programs that teach families about the various stages of Alzheimer's and about ways to deal with difficult behaviors and other caregiving challenges are helpful. Joining a support group has proven to be helpful for certain caregivers. Caregivers may find relief, express concerns, exchange experiences, gain advice, and get emotional comfort in these support groups. Many organizations sponsor in-person and online support groups for people with early-stage Alzheimer's disease and their families. Good coping skills and respite care are other ways that help caregivers handle the stress of caring for a loved one with Alzheimer's disease.

Furthermore, being physically active has both physical and psychological benefits. There are a variety of methods and programs that can assist care-givers, and researchers are constantly looking for new and improved ways to support them. The next chapter discusses several factors that can reduce one's risk of developing Alzheimer's.

8

Prevention

In a time not too long ago, it was once believed that Alzheimer's disease was an inevitable by-product of aging and genetics. If certain markers were observed in genetic tests, or if a person's family history suggested the likelihood of future diagnosis, rarely did people take preventive action to reduce their prospect of developing the disease. After all, Alzheimer's disease has always been known as an unrelenting brain disease with strong genetic loadings. Recall from chapter 5 that no current treatment is effective in stopping the debilitating progression of the disease. In addition, unlike lung cancer or obesity, conditions that can be at least somewhat improved with efforts that are obvious to most patients (eat better, exercise, do not smoke), there have not been many data to indicate which lifestyle changes could be made to slow neurological decline, aside from vague and speculative advice. In those times, an Alzheimer's disease diagnosis offered little hope for patients; it was often viewed as a description of how one should expect to die, and little else. But modern research paints a different, more hopeful landscape involving preventive approaches for Alzheimer's disease. Multiple investigations have shown that for most people, the fate of one's cognitive health is not entirely within one's genes. Although preventive efforts cannot halt the progression of Alzheimer's disease, dementia symptoms and one's quality of life can indeed be improved—sometimes quite significantly—under the right conditions. This chapter will review several measures that have been shown to reduce one's risk of developing Alzheimer's disease. It is important to point out that "reducing risk" is *not* synonymous with prevention. Individuals who take measures to reduce their risk may still develop dementia, but they may be less likely to develop it or may develop it later in life than they would have if they had not taken steps to reduce their risk. Even if you are not at genetic risk for Alzheimer's disease, the topics covered in this section are believed to reduce your risk of cognitive decline—because as we will soon see, genes offer no guarantee that your brain is safe from neurocognitive decline.

GENETICS AND PREVENTIVE MEDICINE

The medical model of treating Alzheimer's disease is all about improving one's quality of life by reducing the frequency, intensity, and duration of Alzheimer's disease symptoms, but unfortunately, no medical procedure or marketed miracle pill can cure Alzheimer's disease. The disease will take the life of a patient within 3 to 20 years after diagnosis, with the average life expectancy between diagnosis and death being 8 to 10 years. We all know people who have survived severe illnesses and medical complications, but when it comes to Alzheimer's disease, there are no survivors. The overall failure of pharmaceutical efforts to reduce Alzheimer's disease has led researchers to investigate the uses of experimental treatment methods (see chapter 10), but most researchers believe that the best way to treat Alzheimer's disease is to use a prophylactic (preventive) approach.

The encouraging outlook offered by prophylactic approaches to managing Alzheimer's disease seems overly optimistic when we read about certain genes that have been found to raise the risk of Alzheimer's disease. Ever since the human genome was mapped in 2003, scientists have known how certain genotypes can be predictive of certain outcomes. But here is where some misinformation can set in. Let's briefly review some basic genetic principles before moving forward.   An important thing to know is that some diseases are caused by *genetic mutations*, which are permanent changes in one or more specific genes. So, if you inherit a disease-causing genetic mutation, then you will likely develop the disease. Huntington's disease, cystic fibrosis, and sickle cell anemia are all examples of inherited genetic disorders caused by gene mutations. However, in other diseases, *genetic variants* may occur. This type of gene change can sometimes cause a disease directly, but more commonly, it serves to increase or decrease a person's risk of developing a certain disorder. Genetic risk factors are defined as genetic variants that increase a disease risk but do not directly cause disease. So is Alzheimer's disease a genetic mutation or a genetic variant? It is both.

Scientists have identified a genetic mutation that usually causes early-onset familial Alzheimer's disease (EOFAD), but this only represents about

5% of all Alzheimer's disease cases. Researchers have not identified a specific gene that causes late-onset Alzheimer's disease. However, one genetic risk factor that appears to increase one's odds of developing late-onset Alzheimer's disease is associated with the apolipoprotein E (APOE) gene on chromosome 19, which contains instructions for building a protein that allows fat and cholesterol to be transported in the bloodstream. Many studies have found that a specific variant of this gene, APOE ε4, is associated with the risk of developing late-onset Alzheimer's disease, but the process of how this occurs is not well understood. Importantly, inheriting the APOE ε4 gene, which is present in 10% to 15% of the population, does not mean that a person will develop Alzheimer's disease. Some people with one or even two APOE ε4 alleles never get the disease, and on the other side of the coin, it is entirely possible to develop Alzheimer's disease without any APOE ε4 alleles at all. And among the tens of thousands of patients whose Alzheimer's pathology has been studied in clinical settings, purely genetic cases are much less common than those linked to environmental and behavioral influences. In sum, it is time to stop categorizing Alzheimer's disease as a genetic inevitability, as research shows that this simply is not the case for about 95% of the population. The focus, then, turns to what we can do to prevent or reduce our chances of developing Alzheimer's disease.

Preventive thinking has been part of many ancient societies, but it has only started to receive scientific attention in the past 30 years. Research on preventive measures for Alzheimer's disease is beginning to skyrocket. As we have seen in previous chapters, many recent studies have suggested that neuropathological change exists in the brain decades before the patient begins to notice symptoms of cognitive decline, but most preventive interventions used by medical professionals are started years or decades after the emergence of Alzheimer's disease symptoms. According to the American Public Health Association, efforts to delay the onset of Alzheimer's disease can be extremely worthwhile: if the onset of symptoms were delayed by as little as 5 years, it would mean for a 50% reduction in Alzheimer's disease rates within 30 years. Although countless research projects have identified a variety of factors that correlate with improvements in managing Alzheimer's disease, perhaps the most substantial and promising results are found within a few key areas: diet, exercise frequency, sleep, cognitive reserve, and stress reduction.

DIETARY FACTORS

Several areas of research suggest that one's diet plays a significant role in the development of Alzheimer's disease. Carbohydrates are an especially pernicious dietary component because when they are consumed in high quantities, they can trigger insulin resistance, which has been shown in several studies to increase one's chances of developing dementia later in life. Here is how it works: when you eat a Snickers bar, a bowl of Special K cereal, or even a slice of whole-wheat toast, your blood sugar levels rapidly increase, because your digestive system quickly converts the high levels of carbohydrates in those foods into glucose, a simple sugar that is used by the body as energy. However, our cells do not simply absorb glucose from the bloodstream. Instead, they rely on insulin, a hormone secreted by the pancreas that allows cells to transport glucose into muscle, fat, and liver cells for energy storage. You might already be familiar with insulin, especially given its key role in diabetes—a disease which ranks as the seventh-leading cause of death in the United States, just below Alzheimer's disease.

Both type 1 and type 2 diabetics have chronic problems maintaining healthy insulin levels, but for different reasons. Type 1 diabetes, which is generally diagnosed in childhood or adolescence, is a lifelong autoimmune condition in which the body's own defense systems mistakenly attack and destroy pancreatic cells that produce insulin, resulting in a dangerous lack of this vital hormone when carbohydrates are consumed. Type 2 diabetes, in contrast, is typically diagnosed later in life and occurs when the pancreas must work especially hard to pump out insulin to reduce chronically high blood sugar levels caused by diets rich in sugar and carbohydrates. By moving blood sugar into cells for storage, insulin allows our blood sugar to return to stable levels. Normal, healthy cells are sensitive to insulin. But when our cells are continually overexposed to insulin, insulin resistance occurs as the body's cells become less responsive to it. The type 2 diabetic may then require increasingly more insulin if healthy blood sugar is to be maintained. Because of problematic insulin levels, both types of diabetics are at risk for developing hyperglycemia (high blood sugar), which wreaks havoc on our heart, kidneys, eyes, and our body's ability to deal with infections. But how is diabetes related to Alzheimer's disease?

Alzheimer's disease also involves problems with insulin. Diets high in sugars and carbohydrates not only affect the body's ability to regulate blood sugar but they also cause negative effects on the brain. If insulin cannot easily enter nerve cells, deficits in memory and learning may be observed. There is a burgeoning amount of research that suggests a strong link between impaired insulin signaling in the brain and cognitive decline. This relationship has been observed since 2005, and it has been so convincingly demonstrated that some researchers have even used the term "type 3 diabetes" to describe Alzheimer's disease pathology. This moniker may seem a bit surprising, but research reveals a shocking statistic: diabetics are twice as likely to develop Alzheimer's disease. But insulin insensitivity may not be the only reason for why diabetes and Alzheimer's disease share such a striking relationship. New York University professor Melissa Schilling has offered another explanation for why diabetes may predict Alzheimer's disease—even among diabetics who successfully reduce their insulin through blood sugar–lowering medications. Schilling hypothesizes that insulin-degrading enzyme, a naturally occurring enzyme responsible for natural insulin degradation in the body, is a key factor because it is also innately used by the body to break down amyloid plaques in the brain. Diabetics who do not form enough insulin may suffer cognitive decline because there is not enough insulin-degrading enzyme to break down these plaques. Even diabetics who take insulin suffer from cognitive decline because their bodies end up with excessive levels of insulin. In their case, most of the insulin-degrading enzyme gets used up breaking down injected insulin, leaving little left over for the decomposition of amyloid plaques in the brain.

Consistent with this hypothesized relationship, a longitudinal Japanese study that tracked 135 people over 10 years found that postmortem amyloid plaques were present among 72% of people who had developed insulin resistance. Even among those who had high blood sugar levels *without* insulin resistance, 62% showed evidence of amyloid plaques in their autopsied brains, further suggesting a worrying relationship between elevated blood sugar levels and the development of Alzheimer's disease. This finding matches up with another report found in the *Journal of Alzheimer's Disease*, which concluded that people who indulge in high-carbohydrate diets (which routinely spike insulin to overwhelming levels), have nearly four times the risk of developing mild cognitive impairment. And for people who have the APOE ε4 genetic variant, making dietary changes to avoid insulin resistance is especially important. A 2018 study found that, among people who tested positive for the APOE ε4 allele, those who were also insulin resistant were 30% more likely to test positive for the presence of amyloid in the brain. This is a staggering finding because it demonstrates that even though you cannot control whether you have the Alzheimer's gene variant, you absolutely *can* control whether you develop insulin resistance, now recognized as an especially important factor for people at genetic risk for Alzheimer's disease.

Reducing your dietary consumption of carbohydrates and sugars is not only recommended if you have a family history of Alzheimer's disease or if you or one of your loved ones has already developed some type of cognitive impairment. If you rely on carbohydrates for 60% (or more) of your diet—as the typical American does—you are putting yourself at risk for insulin resistance, later-life dementia, and several other health conditions. Limiting breads, pastas, cereals, and starches in your diet is one of the best things that you can do for the health of your brain—no matter what type of APOE variant you have.

Further research suggests that additional dietary measures could stave off dementia. We have known for years that diets such as the DASH (Dietary Approaches to Stop Hypertension) and Mediterranean help reduce heart disease and may be able to reduce the risk of dementia as well. The DASH diet aims to reduce blood pressure, while the Mediterranean diet is inspired by the typical diets of people who reside in regions bordering the Mediterranean Sea. Both diets encourage people to eat foods that are low in saturated fat, total fat, and cholesterol, and high in fruits and vegetables. In addition, people should consume whole grains, poultry, fish, and nuts while decreasing their intake of fats, red meats, sweets, sugary drinks, and sodium (e.g., using herbs to flavor food rather than salt). To illustrate the benefits of eating certain fruits, a 2012 study published in the journal of *Annals of Neurology* found that consumption of berries and flavonoids showed a slower rate of cognitive decline in women ages 70 and higher. Flavonoids are antioxidants with anti-inflammatory and immune-system benefits and are found in most fruits and vegetables. Researchers used data from the decades long Nurses' Health Study, which began in 1976. Every four years, the women participants were questioned on their eating habits. Between 1995 and 2001, more than 16,000 women age 70 and older underwent memory testing. The researchers found that greater ingestion of blueberries and strawberries was related to slower rates of cognitive decline for up to 2.5 years. Those who consumed two or more servings of the berries each week showed the most improvement. Why? According to the Alzheimer's Association, berries contain a particularly high number of flavonoids called anthocyanidins, which are capable of crossing the blood-brain barrier and localizing themselves in the hippocampus, an area of the brain involved with memory.

Another relatively recent dietary approach that has shown some benefit for treating Alzheimer's disease is the administration of a ketogenic diet. When a person continuously eats a very low amount of carbohydrate (usually no more than 20 grams per day), the body eventually burns through its main sources of energy: glucose (sugar in the blood) and glycogen (stored sugar in the liver and muscles). This makes the body rely on fat as an alternate source of fuel. The liver begins to produce ketones, also known as ketone bodies, which are a type of acid that is sent through the bloodstream to fuel muscles and other body tissues. As a result of relying on fat for energy, people typically begin to shed extra pounds of fat, which is why the ketogenic diet has recently become a popular dietary trend. As with any extreme-sounding diet, you may think that all of this sounds a bit unnatural or dangerous, but consider: in prehistoric days, when food sources were scarce, ketosis developed as a survival mechanism that built its way into human evolution. Our energy-hungry human brain consumes about 20% of the body's total energy, despite being only 2% of the body's total mass. The ability to transition from burning carbohydrates to burning fat for fuel was necessary for our ancient ancestors, who needed a steady supply of energy to continue hunting and gathering, even though their blood glucose was depleted and their glycogen reserves were exhausted in times of starvation. Mild ketosis is actually a highly natural metabolic state, because for 99.9% of human history, humans did not rely on carbohydrates as a primary energy source. It was only with the dawn of the agricultural revolution that humans shifted their primary diet of proteins and fats to carbohydrate-laden grains, which became a more common source of food because of its wide availability and ease of preservation. And importantly, research shows that ketones protect the brain by enhancing antioxidant protection while suppressing dangerous inflammation. They also decrease free-radical production in the brain, stimulate the development of energy-creating mitochondria, and block a form of programmed neural cell death. A ketogenic diet is not only natural but also incredibly healthy.

Several human research studies have provided evidence that a diet that induces ketosis has beneficial effects for those suffering from dementia. In 2012, University of Cincinnati researchers randomly assigned 23 older adults with mild cognitive impairment (MCI) to either a high- or very low carbohydrate diet for six weeks. At the end of the study, researchers observed many positive health improvements among the very low carbohydrate group, including reductions in weight, fasting insulin levels, and waist circumference. But they also observed a strong relationship between ketone levels and memory performance, suggesting that the ketogenic state was associated with cognitive improvements. However, as anyone who has tried a ketogenic diet will tell you, limiting carbohydrate intake to less than 20 milligrams a day is not easy to do. Other research on the subject examined how sustained levels of mild ketosis, achieved even in the presence of a normal diet with normal amounts of dietary carbohydrates, can improve cognition. Over the course of 90 days, 152 patients who were previously diagnosed with mild to moderate Alzheimer's disease drank a daily ketogenic compound made up of medium-chain triglycerides (MCTs). A comparison group, made up of individuals who were diagnosed with the same types of dementia, ingested a placebo for the same number of days. On average, there was a significant difference between the comparison groups: people who drank the daily MCT compound showed significantly higher improvements on tests of cognition and memory after 45-day and 90-day assessments. This research shows that even in the absence of a full ketogenic diet (which is associated with several physical and mental health benefits), even mild states of ketosis achieved through oral ingestion can be beneficial in improving Alzheimer's disease symptoms. The compound used in this study, Axona, has been approved for the treatment of Alzheimer's disease in the United States.

Although research on the effects of a ketogenic diet for those with the APOE ε4 genetic variant are almost absent in the current literature, a 2019 case study found encouraging results. A 71-year-old female who tested positive for APOE ε4 and mild Alzheimer's disease was put on a 10-week protocol that required a ketogenic diet along with increased physical and mental exercise. After the training protocol was complete, researchers observed a 23% improvement in the patient's cognition and memory, as measured by the Montreal Cognitive Assessment (MoCA), a screening tool used to assess several different aspects of memory and thinking. Researchers concluded that this study, even though extremely limited due to its sample size of just one, "suggest[s] that a ketogenic diet may serve to rescue cognition in patients with mild Alzheimer's disease" and that "for APOE ε4 positive subjects . . . ketogenic protocols extend hope and promise for Alzheimer's disease prevention."

EXERCISE

When you think of how cognitive decline may be prevented in old age, you may assume that doing things to keep your mind active—such as doing daily sudoku puzzles, joining a reading group, or continuing to learn new things—may be the best way to protect against dementia. But surprisingly, research has shown that physical exercise is a better way of increasing your intelligence and reducing your risk of cognitive decline. According to a large brain-imaging study that used magnetic resonance imaging (MRI) to examine the brains of 600 people between the ages of 70 and 73, it was found that as physical exercise increases, brain shrinkage decreases. No such benefit was observed among those who participated in mentally stimulating activities for a period of three years—at least in terms of brain size. Though the study made no strong conclusions about the efficacy of cognitive stimulating experiences, the results were clear—exercise provides a powerful way of shaping the physical structure of the aging brain.

An abundance of research has shown that exercise is absolutely imperative for brain health, cognitive ability, and dementia prevention. Not only does it decrease insulin resistance, which helps prevent diabetes, it also reduces inflammation—a common but potentially deadly biochemical reaction that underlies all degenerative illness, including brain disease (see chapter 10). Exercise also activates codes for brain-derived neurotropic factor (BDNF), a type of protein that supports the survival of existing brain cells and fosters the development of new ones. Interestingly, BDNF encourages connections between nerve cells and is found in abundance in brain areas that are crucial for learning, memory, and complex thought processes. A 2018 study by a Massachusetts General Hospital research team demonstrated that "exercise is one of the best ways to turn on neurogenesis," noting the powerful ability of BDNF to create a hospitable environment for new neurons to survive. The researchers, who investigated Alzheimer's disease in mouse brains, are working on ways of harnessing the power of the exercise-derived neuroprotein for use in future Alzheimer's disease treatments. The researchers believe that one major reason why current pharmacotherapies for Alzheimer's disease do not work very well is that newly generated neurons cannot survive in brain regions that have already been devastated by the progression of Alzheimer's disease. One of the researchers concluded that "the lesson learned was that it is not enough just to turn on the birth of new nerve cells. You must simultaneously 'clean up' the neighborhood in which they are being born to make sure the new cells survive and thrive. Exercise can achieve that, but we found ways of mimicking those beneficial cognitive effects by the application of drugs and gene therapy that simultaneously turn on neurogenesis and BDNF production." How striking—a protein derived from exercise may be the key that allows for future medical treatments to be more effective. Need more proof that exercise offers powerful protection against dementia? Consider this: in 2018, the American Academy of Neurology created a set of recommendations that offered the very best guidelines a doctor could follow in order to properly treat patients suffering from mild cognitive impairment. The subcommittee tasked with coming up with these recommendations exhaustively studied eight potential medications that may prove helpful in treating Alzheimer's disease, but their only meaningful recommendation was that clinicians should recommend exercise as a way of boosting cognitive health.

Exercise is such a powerful factor in treating dementia that it even shows promise for treating people who have genetic markers for Alzheimer's disease. A 2012 study reported in the *Journal of Neurology* tracked the physical activity of over 600 participants for five years and found that a higher level of total daily physical activity was associated with significant reductions in the risk for developing Alzheimer's disease—even among those with the APOE ε4 variant. The study made it clear that frequent daily movement, even at low intensity, can have a meaningful impact on dementia risk reduction—which is good news for those of us who feel overwhelmed even thinking about intense physical exercise. But for those of us willing to put in the extra effort, intensity of exercise offered additional benefits: when examining intensity of exercise, the researchers found that people who engaged in the most physical activity (the top 10%) experienced more than double the risk reduction of Alzheimer's disease in comparison to those who engaged in the least strenuous workouts (the bottom 10%). The message is clear: frequency and intensity of exercise can be powerfully protective. And lastly, what about those who have the rare genetic mutation for early-onset Alzheimer's disease? Is it worth adding an exercise regimen? The answer seems to be yes. A 2018 study found that people who engaged in at least 150 minutes of aerobic exercise per week experienced significantly better cognitive test scores and less tau protein in the brain—and those results held true even for people with genetically driven Alzheimer's disease.

SLEEP

There seems to be a connection between sleep and the formation of brain proteins that are linked to Alzheimer's disease. As nerve cells conduct their regular functions, they leave behind waste products such as amyloid beta, a breakdown of a larger protein that is thought to be important in forming connections between nerve cells and guiding the migration of nerve cells during early development. The role of this larger protein in adulthood is less clear, but when it breaks down in the brain, one by-product, called beta-amyloid 42, is thought to be especially toxic. The body usually clears away amyloid beta, but sometimes, especially when it is sleep deprived, the brain does not get the chance to flush out all of it. Amyloid begins to collect in the junctions between nerve cells of the brain, and if it piles up too much, it can accumulate into plaques that are thought to eventually lead to other problems such as inflammation and the abnormal buildup of tau protein, again, another major biomarker associated with Alzheimer's pathology. Tau appears to destroy neurons if it becomes tangled inside nerve cells. These neurofibrillary tangles block nerve cells' ability to transport nutrients and molecules within themselves, which reduces communication between cells and leads to Alzheimer's disease.

Researchers at the University of Rochester Medical Center in New York have identified how deep sleep may protect against the development of Alzheimer's disease. Their research suggests the presence of a self-cleaning system in the brain that regularly washes away neurotoxins and waste products that accumulate over the course of each day. Known as the *glymphatic system*, this protective mechanism relies on cerebrospinal fluid (CSF), a clear, plasma-like substance located in the brain and spinal cord that receives filtration from the bloodstream. Each night, the glymphatic system activates to ensure that we will awake the next morning feeling refreshed and mentally sharp. But here is the important part: because this system requires a lot of energy to complete, it typically operates only once we have achieved a deep state of sleep. In their 2019 study, Rochester investigators monitored the brains of mice who were put to sleep by means of different chemical injections intended to produce different levels of sleep. It was found that the deeper the drug-induced sleep, the more efficiently the mouse's glymphatic system operated. The same researchers had previously noted how the glymphatic system was successful in removing beta-amyloid and tau from rodent brains—the same biological markers of

Alzheimer's disease seen in humans. It seems that this newly discovered cleaning system is possibly important for the prevention of Alzheimer's disease, and its efficiency is modulated by the quality of one's sleep.

Research on human populations has further linked biomarkers of Alzheimer's disease to sleep disturbance, further suggesting the possible importance of sleep as a preventive measure for reducing risk of Alzheimer's disease. Investigators from the Knight Alzheimer's Disease Research Center conducted a study on 189 cognitively normal participants. Their brains were studied using CSF analysis and/or positron emission tomography (PET) scans, which tracked the presence of amyloid beta. None of the 139 participants showed any evidence of preclinical Alzheimer's disease, and of this group, most had normal sleep-wake cycles. However, the 50 participants who showed positive signs of preclinical Alzheimer's disease, marked by the presence of amyloid in the brain, all reported significant disruptions in their sleep-wake cycle. Even after controlling for age and sex, researchers found a correlation between disrupted circadian rhythms and the presence of amyloid proteins. Although this study and several others like it have found a connection between poor sleep and possible markers of Alzheimer's disease, the direction of causation is unclear, leaving a chicken-or-egg type of problem: Is it that the underlying neuropathology of Alzheimer's disease causes people to get poor sleep, or is it that poor sleep promotes the biological changes in the brain characteristic of Alzheimer's disease?

The research is inconclusive, but there seems to be at least some evidence of causation between poor sleep and the buildup of amyloid and tau in the brain. Research from the Washington School of Medicine, the Radbound University Medical Centre, and Stanford University has concluded that disrupting just one night of healthy sleep results in an increase of amyloid beta, and a week of disturbed sleep results in elevated tau levels. However, the researchers caution against overinterpreting these findings: amyloid and tau levels probably go back down the next time a person has a good night's sleep. The problem occurs when disturbed sleep becomes a chronic problem. As animal studies have demonstrated, this is when amyloid-beta and tau proteins accumulate more consistently and lead to increased risk for Alzheimer's disease.

MENTAL ENGAGEMENT

The old adage "use it or lose it" may hold a particularly strong meaning when it comes to identifying ways to prevent cognitive decline. As we have known since the late 1940s, the human brain demonstrates remarkable plasticity. That is, as a result of experience, the brain is capable of generating new neurons, pruning old and infrequently used connections between cells, forming additional connections between cells, and increasing capillary density to provide additional blood flow to brain regions of high usage. As if this wasn't already fascinating in its own right, it's even more remarkable to consider that this process of neuroplasticity continues to occur throughout the life span, even throughout old age. But how can the power of our ever-changing brain be harnessed to offer better protection against Alzheimer's disease?

The term "cognitive reserve" often appears in the scientific literature about dementia. As discussed in chapter 3, *cognitive reserve* refers to the variation among individuals in terms of their ability to flexibly engage in alternative problem-solving strategies when engaging in a challenging mental task. In simpler terms, think of cognitive reserve as the brain's ability to improvise and shift into high gear when a demanding situation calls for it. Over time, as a person learns to adeptly shift between different modes of mental processing, preexisting neural networks within the brain become more dense, efficient, and robust, allowing the brain to form a protective neural "reserve" against future brain pathology. Additionally, brains with high cognitive reserve may develop alternative neural processing networks, which can help compensate for the diseased disruption of preexisting networks that are characteristic of Alzheimer's disease. Researchers have observed that dementia patients are more likely to develop cognitive reserve if they sustain a high level of cognitive ability throughout their lives. Research suggests that higher levels of mental activity are associated with an approximate 50% reduction in the risk of developing dementia within the next 4 to 5 years, even among those who tested positive for the presence of the APOE4 ε4 gene. However, cognitive reserve cannot stave off the deleterious effects of Alzheimer's disease indefinitely. Researchers typically observe that when people with high levels of cognitive reserve ultimately begin to develop symptoms of Alzheimer's disease, they experience much more rapid decline than their counterparts who do not lead mentally stimulating lives. This is because cognitive reserve allows the brain to sustain functioning for an extended period of time, even as the disease spreads within the brain, until neurological atrophy becomes so pervasive that the brain can no longer support itself. Even still, the neuroprotective properties associated with cognitive reserve provide a compelling reason for people at risk of dementia to especially value life endeavors that have been linked to the development of cognitive reserve, such as lifelong learning, occupational and educational advancement, and making time for social and leisure activities.

STRESS

When we think of stress, we may think of the uncomfortable feelings and racing thoughts that we commonly experience when we become overwhelmed with pressures that come from work, school, or family obligations. But to really understand stress, the importance of managing it across the life span, and its dangerous link to Alzheimer's disease neuropathology, we must view it as more than a purely psychological process. Stress has a strong influence on the human nervous system, and it profoundly influences the structure of many of the components of the brain that become compromised as Alzheimer's disease progresses. Chronic, unrelenting stress has been shown to have deleterious effects on the right hippocampal and orbitofrontal regions of the brain, which shrink in volume if the brain is constantly exposed to a deluge of stress hormones. Meditation and mindfulness, two popular approaches used to reduce stress, have been used as the basis for several clinical studies that have sought to improve the lives of those already diagnosed with Alzheimer's disease or cognitive impairment (see chapter 5). But a separate line of research on nondiseased populations offers surprising insights about how these popular stress-reducing practices offer neuroprotective properties that can reduce the risk of developing Alzheimer's disease.

There is good evidence that meditation and mindfulness, two well-researched methods of stress reduction, may prevent or delay the age-related neuronal changes observed in dementia. Chronic stress typically leads to a measurable loss of gray matter in the hippocampus, a part of the brain that plays an important role in memory. Conversely, meditation practice is associated with larger gray matter volume in the hippocampus. This is consistent with other research findings that show increased brain activity in the hippocampus when a person is practicing meditation or mindfulness exercises, suggesting that these stress relief practices may counteract the harmful neurological underpinnings of dementia. People who participate in mindfulness-based interventions also show beneficial results in other areas of the brain. For example, we know that brain atrophy is a common outcome of advanced aging in normal populations, and it occurs at a more dramatic rate among people diagnosed with Alzheimer's disease, who show significantly greater reductions in cortical volume. However, several research studies have found meditation protects against this significant decrease in cortical thickness as a result of aging. Surprisingly, one study even found that the cortical thickness of 40- to 50-year-old meditators was similar to the cortical thickness observed in a 20- to 30-year-old control group. Cortical thickness is known to decrease with age, but not among people who meditate, which is why neuroimaging results of meditators depict brain images that look, on average, 20 years younger than they really are. Similar findings have been observed in other studies, which have shown that the practice of mindfulness activates brain regions involved in attention regulation, body awareness, and emotion regulation—the same functions that become compromised as Alzheimer's disease progresses. Researchers are not completely sure if engaging in meditation is the cause of these neurological changes. For instance, it could be that people who choose to practice mindfulness may have unique cerebral differences that attract them to mindfulness in the first place, or they have different neural wiring that helps them continue with ongoing practice. But it has been demonstrated that meditation may produce brain growth (neuroplasticity) and preserve the health of brain cells (neuroprotection).

Stress-reduction practices may indeed serve to prevent neurodegeneration, but evidence for the opposite has also been observed: frequent stress can directly influence the development of neurological abnormalities that serve as key biomarkers for the development of Alzheimer's disease. Working with genetically modified mice, researchers at Temple University School of Medicine conducted a series of experimental investigations to determine how stress might be responsible for increasing the presence of tau protein in the brain. The researchers injected mice with high levels of stress hormones each day for one week to mimic the body's response to chronic stress. By the end of the week, the injected stress hormones produced no immediate changes in mouse memory, as measured through their performance in a maze-learning task. However, the researchers noticed significant abnormalities in the brains of the injected mice. Specifically, tau levels were significantly higher in comparison to other mice who did not receive the stress hormone injection. In addition, the stress-injected mice displayed damaged or destroyed synapses. Synapses are junction points between nerve cells where neurons transmit chemical messages, and their increased presence is thought to be one of the strongest biological indicators of learning and memory. The study therefore provided powerful evidence of a causal relationship between stress hormone elevations and two biomarkers that serve as hallmarks of Alzheimer's disease. Even further, the study demonstrated how a week of elevated stress produces worrying changes in brain structure that do not immediately translate into cognitive deficits—but may add up over time before producing a measurable effect on performance. Of course, this is consistent with our current understanding of Alzheimer's disease, which involves the gradual progression of brain abnormality years before cognitive or behavioral symptoms begin to occur. It appears that proper stress management is necessary to stave off these subtle brain changes that could ultimately lead to cognitive decline.

At this point, scientists have conducted many studies on what may work to mitigate the effects of Alzheimer's disease. Although no specific lifestyle change has been shown to effectively reverse the course of disease, there is good evidence that preventive approaches are the best form of resistance that we currently have against neurocognitive decline. It may now be a good time for some self-assessment. What actions can you take now to improve the health of your brain? Are there any changes that you would like to make to your exercise and exercise levels, diet, sleep patterns, stress levels, or mental engagement? If so, what is holding you back?

9

Issues and Controversies

Any public health issue is naturally followed by debate and disagreement, usually because health authorities cannot agree on which approach may offer the best solutions. This is due not only to differences in opinion but also to the fact that many diseases and disorders present multifaceted problems that could potentially be addressed in a variety of ways. This chapter presents several issues and controversies that tend to be universally encountered by patients and families whose lives have been impacted by Alzheimer's disease. The topics presented here have generated much debate among scholars and researchers, whose contrasting viewpoints can allow us to develop some further insights into the complexities of Alzheimer's disease.

DRUG VERSUS NONDRUG APPROACHES

When people are diagnosed with any disease, one of the first questions that comes to mind is, *How can it be cured?* Although there are a variety of medical and psychosocial treatment options available for Alzheimer's disease, it is disappointing that none of them is effective in stopping the deadly spread of brain pathology that underlies a patient's gradually worsening symptoms. It is also discouraging that many of the available symptom management options cannot offer a guarantee that they will actually be effective in reducing the gradually worsening cognitive and behavioral indicators of disease (although symptom relief is a more realistic goal than is seeking a "cure"). Choosing between different treatment options is not an easy task, and careful consideration must be made when choosing the treatment strategy that may best address the patient's unique presentation and life circumstances. For instance, some treatments aim to restore cognitive functioning, while others reduce the behavioral disturbances of the disease, and still others aim to slow the neuropathy of disease progression (with the hope that symptom improvement will follow suit). Nothing about Alzheimer's disease is easy, and there is no clearly delineated treatment path that promises an ideal route to better well-being. Patients, with the help of their physician and their family members, must therefore weigh several treatment options as they consider how to maximize their chance of living comfortably, for as long as possible, in the difficult years the follow an Alzheimer's diagnosis.

A difficult decision about treatment that must be made shortly after diagnosis has to do with the topic of medication, which was last explored in chapter 5. Should a patient begin taking one of the (few) drugs that are available for treating Alzheimer's disease? Or would it be best to use a different, nonpharmacological strategy in order to help the patient improve cognitive function and reduce other troubling symptoms? Although many patients use medications as their primary way to manage the difficulties associated with Alzheimer's disease, there are some reasons why the decision to medicate is sometimes met with hesitation or trepidation. It is generally believed that medications, which target symptom relief at all stages of Alzheimer's disease, are likely to bring benefit to the patients who use them. Supporting this, a landmark 2008 review article from the journal *Alzheimer's Disease & Associated Disorders* found that the effect of all Alzheimer's drugs is statistically significant, which means that they are likely to make a positive impact in helping patients manage their disease. But here's where the controversy will start to become more apparent: the same researchers also concluded that the average benefit of taking these medications seems to be a small one. Only a marginal improvement in cognition and the ability to manage ADLs (eating, bathing, etc.) was observed across multiple studies. Taken together, this evidence suggests that Alzheimer's disease medications are effective for most patients, but they are only expected to cause minor improvements in day-to-day living. Other research has suggested that medications only delay the procession of symptoms by a few months. Of course, any improvement is desirable when a patient is struggling with a debilitating brain disease, but consider this: the same researchers also found that between 30% and 50% of individuals received no benefit at all from their medications. Other studies have shown that the available drugs offer little or no neuroprotection and are effective for only a short duration, as they produce no lasting symptom reduction after the medication is discontinued. But what's the harm in taking them anyway, just to be safe? A few things need to be considered. Medications can be costly, they must be remembered to be taken daily, and as you probably have anticipated, patients are usually concerned about the potential side effects, which can include nausea, diarrhea, vomiting, stomach pain, weight loss, and lack of hunger. All of these things can potentially influence a client's decision to not medicate. But on the other side of the coin, it should be noted that most people who take Alzheimer's disease medications do not typically report such problems. It seems that as many as 20% of patients who take medications will see improvements that are actually better than expected, and for them, the decision to medicate will likely pay off greatly. Unfortunately, there isn't a way to predict how well any particular medication will be tolerated by any particular person, since pharmacological treatments work in tandem with a variety of other genetically determined biochemical factors in order to produce their effects. All things considered, the topic of medication is deserving of its controversial status.

Various nondrug therapies are also available. These options generally aim to improve a patient's quality of life by increasing cognitive abilities, boosting emotional health, and improving independent living skills. These therapies may include cognitive-based interventions (aimed at improving problem-solving, memory recollection, or daily living skills), psychosocial therapies (which build self-esteem, enhance communication, and promote feelings of connectedness), and sensory or stress-reduction therapies (which target the management of behavioral problems associated with dementia, such as anxiety and agitation). Collectively, these approaches are seen as "less risky" than pharmacological treatments, but they are far from ideal. That's because it's often hard to say how useful these common interventions are. Some approaches have received a great deal of study, but others lack any type of high-quality or large-scale research results. Concerns about nonpharmacological treatments often go deeper than their lack of methodological consistency. Although some nonpharmacological approaches may sound safe and easy, it's important to make sure that a chosen intervention doesn't make too many demands of the patient. Treatments must not be viewed as a chore or as a stressful experience; instead, they should offer patients a supportive experience designed to foster a sense of achievement and progress. It could be frustrating for someone with Alzheimer's disease to fail a cognitive task over and over, and even the best efforts to improve memory decline may overwhelm or exhaust the patient. Further, exploring different nondrug treatments may also be time consuming and costly. Because there are many forms of nonpharmacological therapy, it may be a challenge to know which one might offer the best support for a particular patient. That's because determining which therapy is best often requires the help of a range of different specialists to recommend and carry out treatments. Physicians who commonly diagnose Alzheimer's disease are often well trained in prescribing medicine, but they are much less likely to provide nonpharmacological treatments. As a result, the patient will usually need a referral to a specialist (psychologist, social worker, physiological therapist) who may be able to better recommend and carry out a particular nonpharmacological therapy.

Taken as a whole, the best approach to treatment will likely involve a combination of medical and nonmedical interventions for most patients. When it comes to the age-old debate of whether drug or nondrug therapies are best, patients and caregivers must consider the pros and cons offered by both general approaches, and the patient should be involved in the decision-making process as much as possible. The best options will likely involve a careful consideration of the patient's life history, personality, life circumstances, the symptoms the patient finds most distressing, and how far the disease has progressed.

PATIENT AUTONOMY AND END-OF-LIFE DECISION-MAKING

Throughout the course of Alzheimer's disease, most patients want to remain as fully in control of their lives as possible. But as they move through the middle and late stages of the disease, they often lose their ability to determine and communicate their preferences. By the later stages, they will become increasingly incapacitated by advanced cognitive and physical decline and will therefore need to rely on family members to make decisions for them. With this in mind, geriatric professionals commonly suggest that family members adopt a practice of asking patients to describe their "advance directives"—preferences for end-of-life care that are indicated a time when the patient is still able to demonstrate clear thinking and appropriate judgment. Of course, this consideration is made to honor patients' autonomy and to respect their wishes for how they want to live during their final years of life.

The use of advanced directives in Alzheimer's disease allows a patient to communicate important decisions about end-of-life care. For example, if chewing and swallowing become difficult, would a patient prefer to receive food/hydration through a feeding tube? Or if breathing becomes a serious issue, would the patient prefer to use a ventilator? Does the patient want to be sedated near the end of life to live free of pain, albeit in a minimally conscious state? These controversial end-of-life decisions are not easy to make, and they may cause considerable distress for patients to even contemplate, especially given the fact that it is not uncommon for dementia patients to struggle with depression and anxiety. There is a fine line between supporting the autonomy of Alzheimer's disease patients and making them feel overwhelmed with aspects of the end-of-life decision-making process, so the family must determine how much involvement from the patient is best. It may be the case that a cognitively aware patient is unable to consider these topics in enough depth to formulate a clear set of chosen directives. In these cases, family members may have no choice but to compromise the integrity of their relationships with their loved one by making decisions for them, without the patient's input. Families are placed in a similarly difficult position if these topics are not discussed when the patient is cognitively capable of making such decisions.

And furthermore, there is some debate over whether the general idea of soliciting advance directives from a patient is a worthwhile idea in the first place. Some scholars have argued against advance directives, stating that it is impossible for patients to predict how they will want to live when they become incompetent, because as dementia deteriorates the brain more completely, they may experience life in such a radically different way that they may develop a new set of preferences about how they wish to be cared for—preferences that they could not have anticipated without being in a dire state of advanced decline. Proponents of this view have expressed concern that even in extremely late stages of disease, patients may still want to live, and if they could speak, they might express a desired change to their previous decision, which may have been to terminate care when every day becomes a struggle. Others disagree with this view and say that end-of-life decisions must be based on patient directives that were made before their mind became diseased, because not honoring the decisions made by patients in their former, more cognizant state could be seen as a great disregard for a person's autonomy. Another position that attempts to reconcile the two previous viewpoints has suggested that if an advance directive has been made by the patient to terminate life in late stages, this directive should only be honored if the patient shows obvious signs of suffering sadness during the advanced disease state. Of course, these multiple, contrasting perspectives can make it even harder for families to feel that they are making the right decisions about late-stage care, but fortunately, the majority of medical and geriatric professionals are familiar with these ethical struggles and can offer some much-needed guidance and support to families who begin this difficult decision-making process.

TO LIE, OR NOT TO LIE?

When a patient reaches advanced stages of Alzheimer's disease and begins to require full-time care, additional ethical concerns can emerge that stem from the patient's extreme loss of cognitive functioning. During this challenging time, some caretakers may find it easier to avoid sharing certain truths with the patient in an attempt to maintain emotional peace by sacrificing factual accuracy. For instance, patients in the later stages of dementia are known to have significant memory impairment. They often accuse their caretakers of stealing their belongings when they have misplaced them, because acknowledging their own state of cognitive decline may be too difficult for them to accept. This common situation places family members in a bind, because if they confront the patient with what actually occurred, the patient may not believe them and may even develop delusions that can damage the patient-caregiver relationship. Caregivers sometimes recognize that if they accept blame for things that were not their fault, a more peaceful outcome can transpire ("I'm sorry I borrowed your sunglasses. I should have told you."). In this instance, the patient may still be upset but is less likely to develop long-lasting mistrust. A similar situation might involve a severely compromised patient who asks about where a spouse has gone, not remembering that the patient's husband or wife has already passed away. If the caregiver responds truthfully, the patient may experience a considerable grief reaction each time the question is answered, but by lying ("Mary is at the store."), caretakers can avoid such emotional upsets. Some experts believe that lying, when used to maintain the patient's emotional well-being, is justified. Some proponents of this view have even gone as far as to recommend that, if an Alzheimer's patient no longer recognizes a family member, it may be advisable to treat the situation as if it is an initial meeting ("Hi, I'm Matt. It's nice to meet you."). Although this may sound extreme, the rationale behind it is that patients with severe dementia may not recognize family, and instead of making them feel badly by asking them to recall memories that are no longer accessible, a more constructive approach can be best, even if it isn't exactly truthful. But other authorities disagree and state that even in the most challenging situations, caretakers should never lie to patients, because it could easily damage the integrity of the relationship. For example, they prescribe a different solution: redirecting a question to emphasize its emotional significance. These professionals may recommend acknowledging the reality that one's spouse has died, but through careful phrasing that puts the most emphasis on an emotional truth ("I can't believe that it's been ten years since Mary passed away. I miss her every day, but I know she's in peace now. Tell me about your memories of her.") This strategy is not guaranteed to prevent a grief reaction, but it allows for a truthful dialogue that could lessen caregiver avoidance and improve patient emotional well-being—as long as the patient doesn't fixate on the factual reality of the patient's loss. So which approach is best? It's hard to say. The upshot of all this is that when a patient's cognitive abilities worsen significantly, strategies that may lead to the least amount of distress for the caretaker should be carefully considered, as this often translates to less stress for the patient as well. Caretakers will need to examine their own moral compass and the dynamics of their relationship with the patient to determine if, and when, lying can be used to serve a greater good.

This chapter focused on a few of the issues and controversies regarding Alzheimer's disease that pertain to approaches to treatment, end-of- life issues, and how truthful to be as the disease progresses. The next chapter discusses the current prevalence of the disease, methods for diagnosis, and various treatments, and it considers how these may change in the next several years.

10

Current Research and Future Directions

We have come a long way since Alzheimer's disease was first diagnosed over a century ago in 1906, yet there is much that we still do not know about the disease. Uncertainties about its origins still persist, a definitive diagnosis still requires a postmortem confirmation, and a cure remains undiscovered. But at least one thing appears to be certain: as the aging population increases, so, too, will the number of people who are expected to receive an Alzheimer's disease diagnosis. Because the disease represents a looming health crisis, it is imperative for researchers to develop more advanced assessment techniques in order to maximize the efficacy of current and future treatments. At the same time, there is a crucial need for the development of better therapeutics and disease management options. Of course, promising pharmaceutical developments are never far from the news headlines, but despite decades of research and billions of invested dollars, there is no medication or treatment available that effectively ends the devastating progression of Alzheimer's disease—but that may soon change. Let us turn our sights toward the future and examine the ever-changing landscape of Alzheimer's disease research, which will help us envision what the next decade and beyond might look like.

PREVALENCE

As mentioned in chapter 1, the prevalence of Alzheimer's disease refers to the number and proportion of people in a population who are expected to have Alzheimer's disease at a given point in time. Recall that Alzheimer's disease presents the greatest risk for people over the age of 65, so the population of individuals age 65 and older is of particular interest to researchers who study dementia. In 2020, an estimated 5.8 million Americans age 65 and older were living with Alzheimer's disease, according to the *Journal of the Alzheimer's Association.* To put that statistic into perspective, a staggering 10% of people age 65 and older are believed to currently display clinical symptoms that suggest the presence of Alzheimer's disease brain pathology. Although the number of people who are currently affected by the disease has already reached a concerning number, researchers expect to see prevalence estimates rise dramatically over the next several years and decades. For instance, in the year 2025, the number of Americans age 65 and older with Alzheimer's disease is expected to climb to 7.1 million (a 22% increase since 2020). By 2030, disease prevalence is expected to reach 8.4 million, and by 2040, 11.6 million Americans will qualify for a diagnosis. By 2050, the furthest year forecasted by researchers, Alzheimer's disease is expected to affect close to 14 million people living in the United States (assuming there is no breakthrough treatment discovered by then). That's more than twice the number of Americans living with Alzheimer's disease in 2020.

This alarming upward trajectory in projected Alzheimer's disease cases can be explained by the fact that Americans are now living longer than ever before. Today, more and more Americans are living well into their 80s, 90s, and beyond. But as the population of Americans over the age of 65 rapidly grows from 56 million in 2020 to 88 million by 2050, so, too, will the number of people living with Alzheimer's disease. And that's not the only reason for a projected spike in Alzheimer's cases. The proportion of elderly individuals living in the United States is higher than it has ever been—and it is growing. According to 2017 data from the U.S. Census Bureau, adults over the age of 65 now represent as much as 16% of the overall U.S. population—and that proportion is expected to increase to 20% by 2030. The baby boom generation, a large cohort of people born between 1946 and 1964 in the thriving post–World War II economy, has already started to reach age 65 and beyond in increasing numbers. The oldest baby boomers will be 74 years old in 2020, and by 2031, the first baby boomers will reach age 85 and beyond, the age group referred to as the "oldest old." The elderly will become one of the nation's largest populations in the coming years. It is now expected that in 2034, people age 65 and older will outnumber children ages 0 to 18 for the first time.

Although it is widely expected that Alzheimer's disease will rise nationally and globally in the near future, the numerical projections highlighted in the preceding paragraphs are not capable of showing the potentially positive effects that treatment and preventive factors may have in reducing

Alzheimer's disease prevalence in the coming years. All of the aforementioned statistics show an increase in Alzheimer's disease numbers because of the sheer volume of people who will, according to U.S. Census data, enter the 65-and-older category in the next few decades. For this reason alone, Alzheimer's disease will necessarily rise, and this is undisputed. But when researchers look at Alzheimer's disease prevalence over shorter durations and among more specific populations, they are able to observe trends that future national estimates do not incorporate in their predictive models. Interestingly, more than a dozen research studies published over the past decade have suggested that rates of Alzheimer's and other dementias have actually *fallen* between the mid-1990s and today, possibly due to advancements in controlling cerebrovascular risk factors as well as increased opportunities for people to continue their education (which may allow more people to build cognitive reserve; see chapters 3 and 8). The results of these studies offer good news because they provide evidence that the identification and control of potential dementia risk factors is a valuable process. It is unknown whether this encouraging trend in dementia reduction will continue in the foreseeable future, or if it will be undermined by expected worldwide increases in obesity and diabetes, which have been strongly linked to the development of Alzheimer's pathology.

It should be noted that all of the nationwide epidemiological studies discussed in this section have used clinical symptoms (such as memory loss or problem-solving deficiency), and not biomarkers (biological variables suggestive of Alzheimer's disease, such as tau proteins in cerebrospinal fluid [CSF]), in order to diagnose research participants with Alzheimer's disease and ultimately, forecast their predictions about current and future prevalence. When clinical symptoms are used to make diagnosis, there is a potential for "false-positives" to make it into the sample data pool, which could lead to some inaccuracies when making population projections. Interestingly, several research studies have shown that 15% to 30% of people who show clinical symptoms of Alzheimer's disease *do not* actually show the brain pathology necessary to receive a definitive diagnosis of Alzheimer's disease; apparently, these individuals were misdiagnosed, and their dementia symptoms are better accounted for by some other factor or condition. It is therefore most accurate to conclude that the population projections discussed in this section are more likely to predict future prevalence of possible Alzheimer's *dementia*, but not necessarily Alzheimer's *disease*. The alternative, using biomarkers as a diagnostic method in prevalence research, could offer a different way of understanding Alzheimer's disease prevalence. This method would likely result in *lower* numbers of projected Alzheimer's disease cases, because more people show clinical symptoms of probable Alzheimer's dementia than they do biological markers of the disease. However, when biomarkers are used to make diagnoses, it is difficult to discern between Alzheimer's disease and other conditions belonging to the Alzheimer's disease spectrum, such as preclinical Alzheimer's disease and mild cognitive impairment (MCI), which can show the same biomarkers as Alzheimer's disease. In addition, research conducted in 2019 has concluded that biomarkers serve as a poor way of diagnosing Alzheimer's disease, since most people with biologically defined Alzheimer's disease do not possess any observable or reported clinical symptoms.

Overall, it is widely expected that the number of Americans diagnosed with Alzheimer's dementia will double over the next 30 years, thanks to longer life expectancies and the large number of rapidly aging baby boomers who are now becoming part of the 65 and older demographic. However, the currently available projections do not take into account the effects of preventive measures or other variables linked to Alzheimer's disease outcomes, making it impossible to use these projections to track progress made toward reducing the numbers of people living with the disease. Future research on Alzheimer's disease prevalence will need to allow for more clearly delineated projections that separate Alzheimer's disease patients from other closely related (but qualitatively different) diagnostic categories that share the same overlapping symptom of dementia. Fortunately, several new diagnostic technologies are on the horizon that will allow researchers and clinicians faster, more valid ways of assessing Alzheimer's disease.

DIAGNOSTIC METHODS

Dementia will become increasingly more prevalent in the years to come, and when dementia symptoms are present, Alzheimer's disease is the most likely etiology, accounting for an estimated 60% to 80% of cases. But despite the growing commonality of the disease, the diagnostic process remains a challenge, because most clinical evaluations are mixed with considerable uncertainty or are largely inaccessible to most people. As described in chapter 5, Alzheimer's disease is most regularly diagnosed in clinical settings using combined data from cognitive tests, physical assessments, family interviews, and neurological evaluations since these evaluations do not require expensive, complex, or invasive medical procedures to confirm diagnosis. However, studies have shown that doctors using these methods are only 50% to 80% accurate in diagnosing the disease. For instance, cognitive assessments are less capable of distinguishing between normal cognition and Alzheimer's disease, and they also show difficulty differentiating between Alzheimer's disease and MCI, according to a 2020 study.

More advanced diagnostic technologies are currently available, but they are also limited in several ways. Magnetic resonance imaging (MRI) and computed tomography (CT) scans are often used in the diagnostic process, but such technologies do not support a biomarker-based diagnosis of Alzheimer's disease. In contrast, they are more often used to rule out other biological causes that may better explain a patient's cognitive deficits, such as tumor, hemorrhage, or stroke. To really confirm diagnosis, CSF tests can be conducted to measure the presence of abnormal proteins that suggest the presence of Alzheimer's disease. This method allows for a more conclusive, biomarker-based diagnosis, but it is also invasive, painful, and not covered by insurance providers. Some other state-of-the-art biomarker-detection technologies are available today to aid in the diagnostic process, such as amyloid positron emission tomography (PET) and single-photon emission computed tomography (SPECT). These nuclear imaging methods allow for accurate detections of Alzheimer's disease biomarkers, but their clinical utility is limited for similar reasons: the assessments typically cost upward of $5,000 to conduct, the cost is not covered by health-care insurance, and both methods require the patient to be injected with a radioactive tracer chemical. Therefore, these advanced technologies are much more widely utilized in research settings than in real-world clinics.

Another glaring limitation to current diagnostic methods is that they are usually conducted only when individuals suspect that they may already be experiencing symptoms of dementia. Most Alzheimer's disease diagnoses are made at the early stage, when a person begins to notice that memory is starting to decline and interfere with daily life; however, Alzheimer's disease neuropathology is believed to begin in the brain as many as 15 to 20 years before symptoms emerge. A timely diagnosis of Alzheimer's disease is crucial, because treatments and preventive measures are known to be more effective if they are utilized early in the course of the disease. Recall from chapter 5 that the diagnostic stage of preclinical Alzheimer's disease is suggested when there is biomarker evidence for Alzheimer's disease neuropathology, even though the patient remains asymptomatic. Interestingly, the diagnosis of preclinical Alzheimer's disease is currently meant to be used for clinical research or trials, not in general clinical practice. Although it is presently unknown how many people who qualify for a preclinical Alzheimer's disease diagnosis will progress to MCI or dementia within their lifetime, many researchers have emphasized that the preclinical stage of Alzheimer's disease should be defined as part of the disease process and that this stage should be identified and targeted for treatment soon as possible. Two gold-standard methods are currently available for detecting preclinical Alzheimer's disease, which include the amyloid beta–detecting PET scan and the CSF assay. Both methods successfully detect the characteristic biomarkers of preclinical Alzheimer's disease, amyloid-beta load, and neurodegeneration, but they are each limited in a few key respects: PET scans are expensive, invasive, and largely unavailable for use outside of research settings; CSF assays are subject to significant instrumental error across laboratories and require a painful lumbar puncture (a "spinal tap").

Simpler, safer, and more accessible detection methods are necessary in order to identify the earliest indicators of Alzheimer's disease neuropathology. Scientists are currently working on developing new assessment methods that could shape the future of Alzheimer's disease diagnosis by making the process more accurate, less expensive, and more widely accessible—with a strong focus on identifying preclinical stages of disease. Several novel diagnostic methods are being developed for clinical use, including blood tests, retina imaging, and artificial-intelligence-powered assessments.

Blood Tests

Researchers believe that blood tests might soon offer an inexpensive and widely available method of diagnosing Alzheimer's disease. In 2019, scientists at the Washington University School of Medicine discovered that beta-amyloid sampled from blood plasma could provide a reliable indicator of whether the same sticky protein also existed in the brain, which could confirm the biological presence of Alzheimer's disease. Using an analytical chemistry technique called mass spectrometry, the researchers were able to precisely measure beta-amyloid in the blood of 158 cognitively normal volunteers in their 60s and 70s. Next, the researchers compared each participant's blood level of beta-amyloid to PET scan data that were collected from each participant over the course of several years, which tracked the same amyloid biomarker. Impressively, the researchers found that the blood test was capable of detecting amyloid beta an average of four years before evidence of it appeared in PET scans—which is impressive because PET scan technology is thought be one of the most sensitive methods of detecting evidence of Alzheimer's disease available today. And when the researchers combined these data with other known predictors of Alzheimer's disease—such as age and whether or not participants tested positive for the apolipoprotein E (APOE) ε4 gene—Alzheimer's disease could be detected with a remarkable 94% accuracy, even in patients who did not show any clinical symptoms of the disease. Researchers expect that the blood test will be used in the future to screen people for clinical trials of drugs that could be used to prevent Alzheimer's disease, but they also acknowledged an important limitation: the presence of amyloid beta in the brain does not necessarily guarantee a diagnosis of Alzheimer's disease.

The so-called amyloid hypothesis, which links Alzheimer's disease to brain plaque, has been called into question in recent years by some scientists who are beginning to think that it is possible that tau protein tangles in the brain might be a more direct and accurate marker of Alzheimer's disease neuropathology. With this in mind, a different group of international researchers at the University of California San Francisco developed a different type of blood test in 2020 that could also be used to detect a form of tau protein. This tau protein–based blood test also demonstrated impressive results: it was found to be equally accurate as the more complex and costly PET scan detection method. And further, the same researchers found that the blood plasma–based tau detection method could accurately distinguish Alzheimer's disease from frontotemporal lobar degeneration, a different form of dementia that researchers have previously struggled to differentiate from Alzheimer's disease, especially among relatively younger patients who experience milder symptoms. Impressively, the test was also sensitive enough to predict which patients were cognitively normal and which had MCI. This is all very exciting, because some Alzheimer's disease researchers have referred to blood-based Alzheimer's disease diagnostics as the long-sought-after "holy grail" that could lead to much better Alzheimer's disease screening tools. According to Eliezer Masliah, director of the Division of Neuroscience at NIH's National Institute on Aging, it is believed that blood tests are only a few years away from use in clinical or office settings.

Saliva Tests

A separate line of research has evaluated whether an even less invasive test, one that requires only a small saliva sample, could be used to successfully detect biomarker evidence of Alzheimer's disease. Researchers have recently discovered that most blood biomarkers present in the bloodstream can also be found in saliva. And more directly, specific Alzheimer's disease biomarkers have been shown to migrate down from the brain and spinal cord to the salivary glands, which produce saliva and additional Alzheimer's disease biomarkers of their own. A 2019 systematic review found that that the salivary presence of biomarker *beta-amyloid 42* (Aβ42) appears to be a good candidate for detecting Alzheimer's disease. Using a specific method of biochemical analysis called enzyme-linked immunosorbent assay (ELISA), researchers found that Alzheimer's disease patients had Aβ42 levels that were two to three times higher in comparison to healthy controls, suggesting that salivary levels of the biomarker may be used to predict Alzheimer's disease brain pathology in the future.

Other saliva-based biomarkers were less convincingly detected in populations of Alzheimer's disease patients, mainly because very few research studies have investigated the topic in general, and among those that have, few have investigated biomarkers other than beta-amyloid proteins. However, some inconclusive yet encouraging research has suggested that future saliva-based tests could work by detecting other biochemicals that are known to correlate with Alzheimer's disease neuropathy. For instance, some researchers have noted that the neurotransmitter acetylcholinesterase (AChE), a brain chemical that is known to drop as a result of Alzheimer's disease neuropathology, was significantly lower in Alzheimer's disease patients in comparison to a population of healthy controls, as reported in one of the few studies that investigated this particular biomarker. Other researchers have focused on lactoferrin, a multifunctional iron-binding protein that is found in several body fluids (such as saliva, milk, tears, and nasal secretions) is believed to be another potential indicator of Alzheimer's disease—even though the exact way that this protein affects disease pathology is not well understood. Using ELISA, a 2017 study found that, in comparison to healthy individuals, Alzheimer's disease and MCI patients showed decreased levels of lactoferrin in their saliva samples. The same study uncovered a predictive relationship between lactoferrin and CSF levels of Aβ42 and t-tau, suggesting that the salivary protein could possibly reflect the presence of several other well-studied biomarkers commonly believed to directly indicate the presence of Alzheimer's disease pathology.

One recent study that was not included in the 2019 review investigated whether saliva tests are robust enough to differentiate between people with Alzheimer's disease, MCI, and normal cognition. Using a powerful mass spectrometer that examined more than 6,000 metabolites, substances in the body made when the body breaks down compounds (including its own tissues), researchers found three specific metabolite biomarkers that could successfully distinguish between the three populations of interest, especially when combined with data from processing speed and memory performance assessments. Even though the researchers caution that these results came from a single study with a low sample size, they remain optimistic that saliva tests could one day become a routine part of medical examinations. All in all, because saliva tests are so easy to collect, they can potentially be used as a standard screening tool that becomes part of a future medical checkup routine. Even if future saliva tests may not allow for a conclusive Alzheimer's disease diagnosis on their own, they can potentially be used to indicate when a doctor should prescribe more advanced testing, which can lead to an earlier diagnosis and allow patients more time to implement risk-reduction protocols (see chapter 8).

Retinal Imaging

Long-known as the "windows to the soul," the eyes contain a light-sensitive tissue called the retina. The retina covers the back layer of the eyeball and exhibits characteristics similar to those of the brain, because it develops from the same embryonic cells as the rest of the central nervous system. Many research studies have shown that cellular changes in the retina follow the same changes that happen in the brain, which is not surprising because the retina and the brain share the same neuronal cell layers, blood barriers, complex biochemistry, and neurotransmitter systems. The optic nerve, which directly connects the retina to the cortex, directly transports the compound called amyloid precursor protein (APP) to the brain after it is formed by the retinal ganglion cells. For these reasons, researchers have believed for at least two decades that the retina holds promise as a future diagnostic marker for Alzheimer's disease. But vast improvements in retinal-imaging techniques have emerged since 2010, and high-resolution retinal-imaging technologies such as optical coherence tomography (OCT), blue-light autofluorescence (BAF), and scanning laser ophthalmoscopy (SLO) have made it possible for researchers to precisely examine the retina and explore how it could serve as a "window" to the brain.

Clinical research on human participants has shown that retinal abnormalities can reflect Alzheimer's disease symptoms and neuropathology. In the early stages of Alzheimer's disease, cognitive-visual changes typically manifest, and patients report difficulty with several perceptual abilities, such as reading, finding objects, recognizing and discriminating between colors, identifying the structure of moving objects, and perceiving contrast. Researchers initially believed that these visual deficits were due to the brain degeneration that characterizes Alzheimer's disease, but it is now believed that these abnormalities are due to structural changes that take place within the retina. Postmortem examinations of Alzheimer's disease patients regularly demonstrate evidence of optic nerve degeneration and retinal ganglion-cell loss, and now, thanks to advances in retinal-imaging technology, researchers have observed a few telltale abnormalities in the retinas of living Alzheimer's disease patients. For instance, several researchers have observed a progressive thinning of the retinal nerve fiber layer (RNFL) in Alzheimer's disease patients, and previous meta-analytic research has concluded that retinal thinning can be used as a reliable indicator of Alzheimer's disease neurodegeneration. Further, meta-analyses of studies performed on patients diagnosed with MCI suggest that retinal thinning might also occur to a lesser extent than in Alzheimer's disease–diagnosed patients. Although only a few studies have investigated an association between retinal thinning and lower cognitive scores, a two-year longitudinal study conducted in 2016 found that worse Clinical Dementia Rating and memory competitive scores predicted greater amounts of retinal thinning. Interestingly, the same researchers also found significantly reduced retinal thickness among MCI patients who later developed Alzheimer's disease in comparison to those whose symptoms never worsened.

In addition to retinal thinning, other structural changes in the retina may serve as indicators of Alzheimer's disease. The macula, a portion of the eye at the center of the retina that is characterized by its high density of retinal ganglion cells, decreases by as much as 25% in Alzheimer's disease patients, according to postmortem retinal tissue analyses. Recent studies using optical coherence tomography (OCT), a technology that produces high-resolution cross-sectional scans of the retina, have found that the macula is reduced in Alzheimer's disease patients in comparison to age-matched controls. Consistent with this finding is the observation that macular retinal degradation is less common among MCI populations, who have not yet developed the same symptoms or brain-related neuropathology as Alzheimer's disease patients. There is also evidence that decreased vasculature of the retina may serve as an additional predictor of Alzheimer's disease brain pathology. Disruptions in cerebral vasculature (such as reduced cranial blood flow, hemorrhaging, and infarcts) are common among Alzheimer's disease patients. Because the retina and the brain share so many anatomical and physiological similarities, alterations in the retinal vasculature may reflect the same cerebrovascular pathology that is regularly observed in the brains of autopsied patients.

Retinal imaging shows good potential as a way to identify Alzheimer's disease pathology years before clinical symptoms emerge, but because of several limitations, it may be some time before it becomes available as a diagnostic modality. Very few studies have utilized a within-subjects longitudinal design, a type of research approach that tracks the same individuals over an extended period of time, and therefore, little is known about how the retina changes as one progresses through the different stages of Alzheimer's disease. Another weak point is that the majority of retinal-imaging studies have focused primarily on participants with advanced disease pathology, making it difficult to make retina structure comparisons between control, preclinical, MCI, and mild Alzheimer's disease populations. And because retinal-imaging studies that investigate Alzheimer's disease are only in their infancy, the existing research is marred by studies with low samples sizes and inconsistent instrumentation. Different types of OCT devices built by different manufacturers have been used across different Alzheimer's disease research laboratories. Because of this lack of standardization, image acquisition methods and post-processing algorithms have not been consistently used in the available literature.

Moreover, frequent software updates to OCT systems have been known to modify the ways that the machinery detects neuronal cell edges, making it possible for different research teams to draw different conclusions even if they were to observe the same clinical data.

Even with its shortcomings, retinal imaging offers some exciting possibilities for the future of Alzheimer's disease because of its potential for a convenient, accessible, and affordable biomarker-based diagnosis. Consider the fact that most adults over the age of 50 experience *presbyopia*, a type of farsightedness that develops as the lens of the eye becomes less elastic due to aging. Due to the widespread nature of this condition, it is no surprise that many older adults will periodically visit their eye care specialist in order to update their prescription for corrective lenses. This allows for a convenient opportunity to provide a routine checkup for biological indicators of Alzheimer's disease. Interestingly, optometrists and ophthalmologists are increasingly incorporating advanced OCT retinal-imaging systems into their day-to-day eye office practices, allowing for a more widely available and inexpensive way of collecting biomarker data. Like blood and saliva tests, it is unknown whether retinal imagery will one day become advanced enough to allow for a definitive diagnosis on its own, without the need of additional diagnostic information. However, the method already holds good potential as a low-cost, readily accessible, non-invasive screening tool that could be especially useful in identifying pre-clinical Alzheimer's disease, perhaps in conjunction with an assessment of known risk factors (family history, age, diet, genetic testing results) and other non- or minimally invasive assessments.

TREATMENTS

Pharmaceutical Approaches

There are currently hundreds of drug trials taking place around the world as part of a global initiative to identify new medications and treatments for Alzheimer's disease. Even though no new drug has been recognized by the Food and Drug Administration (FDA) as a clinically effective treatment since the introduction of memantine (Namenda) in 2003 (see chapter 5), there is abundant hope that we will see breakthrough advances within the next decade that address the underlying pathology of the disease in order to stop or limit its progression. According to a February 2020 drug development pipeline report from the Alzheimer's Association, there are 121 products that are currently being tested in clinical trials, which are research studies that thoroughly examine the efficacy and safety profiles of various in-development drugs. Twenty-nine pipeline drugs have advanced to Phase III status, which means that they have demonstrated sufficient results from earlier studies, allowing them be examined on a large-scale basis in order to see if the potential drugs are any better than the pharmaceuticals that are already on the market for treating the same condition or disease. Phase III is the final testing stage needed before a drug is allowed to be submitted to the FDA for final review.

New medications are currently being developed that address at least four different biological pathways that Alzheimer's disease is believed to originate from: senile plaque deposits (composed of amyloid beta, Aβ), neurofibrillary tangles (p-tau), inflammation of the nervous system's immune cells (microglia), and dysfunctions of the 5-HT6 receptor (serotonin). Researchers have not come to a consensus on which treatment strategy will likely be most effective in slowing down or ending cognitive decline. However, regardless of which biological pathway is targeted, it is widely believed that future pharmaceuticals will be maximally effective if they are delivered as early as possible to at-risk groups, further underscoring the importance of a preclinical diagnosis. The efficacy of several therapeutic medications are currently being investigated in clinical trials, with results expected in the early to mid-2020s.

The amyloid hypothesis suggests that the increased production of amyloid beta, specifically the toxic Aβ subtype, serves as the primary cause and the earliest indicator of Alzheimer's disease. This idea has been supported by several studies that have concluded that amyloid beta can be detected in the brain up to 20 years before the onset of clinical symptoms. Researchers have already developed a thorough understanding of how amyloid beta is formed: APP, found in high amounts at the junction point between neurons, is broken down by two enzymes: *beta secretase* and *gamma secretase*. These enzymes break down APP into three fragments, one of which is the peptide amyloid beta. In a healthy state, these protein fragments would be further broken down and eliminated by the body, but in Alzheimer's disease, amyloid beta forms protein clumps known as senile plaques, which are believed to damage and destroy nerve cells. Future medications are being designed to target nearly every possible point in the biochemical pathway that leads to the formation of amyloid beta. One therapeutic that is currently in development, CAD106, works by stimulating the production of antibodies to reduce levels of the harmful plaques, while at the same time preventing the body's autoimmune response, which would otherwise cause cellular inflammation. Another drug in development that aims to reduce amyloid beta is CNP520, which works by preventing the *beta-secretase* enzyme from cleaving the APP precursor protein, thereby reducing the formation of beta-amyloid. Both of these drugs, CAD106 and CNP520, are currently being investigated in prevention studies called GENERATION 1 and GENERATION 2, which have collectively recruited 2,340 cognitively normal individuals, ages 60 to 75, who have all inherited two copies of the APOE ε4 gene (one from each parent). The goal of both studies is to see if the drugs are successful in delaying the time it takes a preclinical patient to reach an MCI or Alzheimer's dementia diagnosis. Both studies are expected to conclude in 2025.

During the writing of this book, the FDA approved a new medication to treat Alzheimer's Disease. Aducanumab (Aduhelm) is the first new therapy to receive FDA approval in almost two decades. This drug is an antibody that is engineered to stick to amyloid-beta molecules in the brain. After the antibody comes in contact with amyloid beta, the body's immune system identifies amyloid beta as a foreign invader, and it is removed from the patient's nervous system. Patients receive the drug intravenously once a month. Clinical trials have showed evidence that Aducanumab successfully reduces amyloid-beta plaques in the brain, and this reduction is assumed to slow down the progression of cognitive decline. This is very exciting news; however, the FDA has required the maker of the drug, Biogen, to conduct postapproval studies to verify that the drug actually produces its intended clinical effect of reducing the rate of cognitive deterioration. These follow-up trials have yet to be conducted and are expected to take place over the next several years. The FDA will continue to monitor the drug, and if it does not work as intended, it will be removed from the market. Also, there is a concern about the cost of the drug. It is estimated that the list price of the drug would be over $50,000 per year of treatment. Only time will tell if this new therapy will be the first to slow the progression of the disease in those living with Alzheimer's.

Future medications are also being developed to target tau protein, another molecule that plays an important role in the pathophysiology of Alzheimer's disease. Predominantly found in neurons, tau protein assembles and stabilizes microtubule structures located inside nerve cell bodies, which allow the cells to maintain their shape and structural integrity. High levels of amyloid beta are believed to trigger hyperphosphorylation of tau protein, an abnormal biochemical process that occurs when phosphate groups excessively combine with tau protein and change its chemical structure. When hyperphosphorylated tau accumulates inside of brain cells, it forms neurofibrillary tangles, twisted fibers within the cell that collapse microtubule structures, leading to neuronal injury and widespread neurodegeneration. ADDvac-1 is a vaccine currently in development that is designed to stimulate an immune system response so that the body's own antibodies can be directed to attack and destroy phosphorylated tau. Researchers are hopeful that the drug will remove phosphorylated tau in the brain, reduce the presence of neurofibrillary tangles, and stop the spread of neuropathology throughout the brain, thereby preventing cognitive decline. Preliminary results of ADDvac-1 showed that 98.2%

of participants who were given the drug successfully generated antibodies to the tau protein, and no adverse effects were observed. Many other tau-mediated drugs are also in development, and several have shown encouraging results in terms of safety and clinical efficacy in animal and human populations, leading researchers to believe that the approach holds significant promise for future drug development.

Recently, there has been a push to develop new therapeutics that may reduce Alzheimer's disease symptoms by addressing the process of neuro-inflammation. As amyloid beta and phosphorylated tau accumulate in the brain, their presence correlates with increased levels of activity in cells called microglia, which guard and protect the nervous system from infections. Microglia are able to move toward areas of the brain where amyloid-beta peptides aggregate, and they can successfully remove amyloid beta in its small, nonaggregate form. However, these protective cells do not have the ability to remove larger senile plaque deposits, and as they interact with these insoluble deposits, microglia initiate a robust inflammatory response. Inflammation plays an important role in the progression of Alzheimer's disease because it predicts detrimental processes like amyloid-beta clumping, neuronal loss, and cognitive deficits. However, the general process of inflammation is not necessarily a bad thing—it is necessary to help the body react and cope with injury or infection. Unfortunately, this immune response sometimes occurs at times when it shouldn't, and the process can be detrimental if it occurs over an extended period of time, as it does in Alzheimer's disease and in other pathologies of the nervous system. With this in mind, anti-inflammatory drugs are being studied for their potential ability to treat Alzheimer's disease. Sargramostim, a drug that has been approved by the FDA to stimulate bone marrow development in patients diagnosed with leukemia, is currently being tested in a Phase II study. The drug works by reducing microglial overactivity, and therefore, it halts brain inflammation. In addition, Sargramostim stimulates microglia and macrophages, white blood cells found in all body tissues, so that they begin to "eat" amyloid-beta fragments, removing them from the brain before they have a chance to aggregate, thereby slowing or stopping Alzheimer's disease progression.

Yet another proposed origin of Alzheimer's disease involves the manipulation of the 5-HT6 receptor, a serotonin molecule receiver found most abundantly in brain areas important for learning and memory. Serotonin receptors are commonly targeted by drugs that are designed to reduce symptoms of depression and anxiety, but those medications affect a different subtype of serotonin. When the areas on a neuron meant to receive serotonin 5-HT6 are blocked by receptor antagonist drugs, a downstream effect occurs, and the brain ultimately begins to produce more acetylcholine (ACh), a neurotransmitter chemical that is known to be low among people living with Alzheimer's disease. Restoring this important neurotransmitter to adequate levels is associated with improvements in memory, attention, and cognition. Notably, 5-HT6 antagonist drugs are meant to serve as a symptom management treatment for Alzheimer's disease, that is, the medications are not expected to stop the progression of the disease, but they might make living with it more tolerable, especially for people who experience behavioral or psychotic symptoms that accompany cognitive decline. Several drug candidates have been developed in recent years that have targeted the 5-HT6 receptor, and although many of these drugs were successful in improving cognition in Phase II studies, they did not show clinical efficacy in the larger and more rigorous Phase III clinical trials. Despite this disappointment, researchers are continuing to investigate this class of treatment with the expectation that more promising results will come from it in the future, when the role of serotonin in Alzheimer's disease is better understood.

Although the past two decades have marked a significant era in terms of understanding Alzheimer's disease, there has been an overall lack of success in developing drugs that significantly minimize or end its devastating progression. This is mostly due to the fact that there are several complex biological pathways that could explain the origin of disease, and each pathway can initiate neurodegeneration independently from the others. In addition, most drugs being clinically tested have shown difficulty crossing the blood-brain barrier, a capillary network surrounding the brain that blocks foreign molecules from entering the central nervous system. And further, the majority of drugs currently undergoing clinical trials work by either targeting the insoluble amyloid-beta plaques that exist outside of neurons or by targeting intracellular neurofibrillary tangles, made up of insoluble tau proteins. But researchers have noted that amyloid-beta and tau proteins are actually produced inside of neurons, where they aggregate and become soluble, toxic oligomer molecules. Most studies suggest that these molecules are the primary culprits in Alzheimer's disease (not the insoluble amyloid plaques or neurofibrillary tangles). Therefore, some researchers believe that future drugs will need to be designed to penetrate neurons so that aggregates of amyloid beta and hyperphosphorylated tau proteins can be dissolved from within nerve cells; however, this has presented a great challenge. For these reasons, researchers believe that a successful pharmacological treatment will need to address several biological variables simultaneously, using a combined treatment approach similar to the ones used to treat cancer and human immunodeficiency virus-1 (HIV). It may be several years or decades before researchers discover a drug that successfully cures Alzheimer's disease, but fortunately, pharmaceuticals may only represent one of several future treatment options.

Novel Nonpharmacologic Approaches

Most research on Alzheimer's disease treatment has explored pharmacological mechanisms aimed at altering a patient's neurochemistry. But a growing number of cutting-edge studies have suggested that a future breakthrough may come out of an entirely different approach—one that utilizes a form of electrical stimulation to reduce Alzheimer's disease symptoms and neuropathology. Researchers are turning their attention to novel, high-tech innovations that are beginning to make it harder to distinguish between science and science fiction. We will now turn our attention to some of the latest advancements that may soon change how we envision the future of Alzheimer's disease treatment.

A wearable, noninvasive headset device for in-home treatment has shown good promise in restoring cognitive function and enhancing memories. The headset utilizes what is known as transcranial electromagnetic treatment (TEMT), which applies an electromagnetic field that penetrates brain cells in order to break up aggregated amyloid-beta and tau protein. After demonstrating that the technology was effective in reversing memory impairment in aged Alzheimer's diseased mice, the first clinical trial was conducted on human participants in 2017. Over a two-month course of treatment, eight human participants who had been previously diagnosed with mild to moderate Alzheimer's disease were given twice-daily 60-minute TEMT treatments that took place in their homes under the supervision of their caretakers. Participants returned to the research clinic periodically so that researchers could measure treatment progress using cognitive tests and CSF biomarker measurements. Cognitive test results showed a large and clinically significant improvement, which was maintained two weeks after treatment was terminated, and a significant reduction in amyloid and tau in a CSF biomarker analysis. Using MRIs, researchers also found evidence of increased communication between neurons in a brain area important for cognition, called the cingulate cortex. No negative side effects were observed, and all participants reported favorable experiences. The company that designed the headset, NeuroEM Therapeutics, is currently conducting subsequent trials on 150 Alzheimer's disease patients in mild to moderate stages of decline, and if successful, the company plans to pursue FDA clearance. However, despite these exciting results, it may be too early to say that the technology offers a breakthrough for Alzheimer's disease, simply because many new treatments have shown remarkable results in early testing, only to fail during later Phase III clinical trials. Researchers remain optimistic that the technology will one day become a standard part of the treatment regimen for Alzheimer's disease.

The future of Alzheimer's disease treatment may also involve a more direct method of stimulating the brain in the form of a neural implant, which may soon offer Alzheimer's disease patients a new way to manage their symptoms and reduce functional decline. In a landmark study conducted in 2017 by researchers at the Ohio State University Medical Center, researchers were the first to demonstrate efficacy of a "brain pacemaker" device, which requires a permanent, surgical insertion of electrical wires into the frontal lobes of a patient's brain. Widely understood as the "command center" of the brain, the frontal lobes govern cognition in the form of, for example, problem-solving skills, organizational abilities, planning, and judgment. By stimulating this brain region using an electrical implant, researchers were successful in helping patients improve their decision-making and problem-solving skills, which are necessary for completing daily living tasks (like making breakfast, retrieving the mail, or socializing with friends or family). Although the technology is not designed to restore a person's loss of memory, it could play a unique role in treating Alzheimer's disease by markedly improving a patient's quality of life, especially as the burden of disease makes independent functioning progressively more difficult. According to Dr. Douglas Scharre, coauthor of the study and director of the Division of Cognitive Neurology at Ohio State's Wexner Medical Center, "We have many memory aids, tools and pharmaceutical treatments to help Alzheimer's patients with memory, but we don't have anything to help with improving their judgments, making good decisions, or increasing their ability to selectively focus attention on the task at hand and avoid distractions." The pilot study showed favorable results, but it was limited to only three participants (for obvious reasons, it is somewhat challenging to get participants to agree to receive a brain implant). However, researchers hope that more robust outcome data will soon follow. Fortunately, advances in this treatment area may come sooner than one might expect, since deep brain stimulation is not an entirely new concept; over the past two decades, it has received significant attention from researchers who have used similar brain implants to successfully treat more than 135,000 Parkinson's disease patients worldwide. Interestingly, other researchers have recently invented a version of the technology that could help Alzheimer's disease patients restore their memory by placing an electrical implant into an area of the brain called the fornix, which plays a key role in learning and memory. In October 2020, medical researchers launched what will be a four-year international Phase III trial to investigate the clinical efficacy of improving memory through deep brain stimulation of the fornix. It should be emphasized that no form of deep brain stimulation has yet indicated the ability to stop the progression of Alzheimer's disease, but researchers plan to explore this possibility further in the Phase III trial. There is some indication that stimulating the fornix could lead to "reawakened" brain activity, which might slow or stop the characteristic atrophy that is so commonly seen in the shrunken brains of Alzheimer's disease patients. Currently, deep brain stimulation looks like it will show the most promise for Alzheimer's disease patients over the age of 65 who are in the early to middle stages of cognitive decline.

Yet another future treatment frontier was conceptualized by a team of investigators from the Massachusetts Institute of Technology (MIT), who examined how flashing lights and sound can be used to generate a brain-wave pattern associated with marked reductions in amyloid-beta and tau protein. Brain waves, in this context, refer to rhythmic patterns of electrical activity generated by neurons that fire at the same frequency. Just as different TV and radio stations are transmitted by different radio wave frequencies, specific brain-wave frequencies are associated with specific neurological functions. A particular type of brain wave relevant to Alzheimer's disease is a gamma wave, which is typically observed when a memory is encoded or stored. This brain wave occurs less regularly in the brains of people diagnosed with Alzheimer's disease, leading researchers to suspect that it may play a role in treatment. The MIT researchers observed that by using specific frequencies of sound and flickering light, they could increase gamma waves in a rodent brain, which triggered a dramatic response in microglial cells. These cells regularly fail in their ability to protect the brain from amyloid plaques, but the gamma waves seemed to galvanize the microglia to respond in a unique way that resulted in a notable reduction in amyloid plaques and tau protein tangles. And moreover, the treated mice showed signs of reduced difficulty in learning how to navigate a maze. Other research groups are now starting to take this idea further by examining whether similar brain-wave manipulations could cause reductions in Alzheimer's disease neuropathy in human Alzheimer's disease patients. More evidence of an effect is certainly needed before any conclusions are made, but researchers speculate that the technology could one day migrate to a smartphone app if it shows clinical promise in clinical trials, and that it may be further conceptualized as a preventive measure, used by middle-aged populations to preserve their cognitive health as they age and become more vulnerable to cognitive decline.

Other areas of research imagine additional ways that Alzheimer's disease can be treated in the years to come, using innovative technologies that address the shortcomings of current pharmacological interventions. One new area of focus explores how a microbubble ultrasound technique can be used to temporarily open the blood-brain barrier, which could allow drug molecules access to the brain. This technique is imagined as a way to solve an important hurdle that severely limits the efficacy of current Alzheimer's disease medications. The technique, pioneered in 2018 by researchers at Sunnybrook Health Sciences Center, involved injecting lipid microbubbles into the bloodstream. When the microbubbles reached the blood-brain barrier near an amyloid-rich area of the frontal lobe, a low-frequency ultrasound wave was applied. This pulse of energy causes the microbubbles to expand and contract, while also allowing them to gently press against the capillary walls and open them up without causing tissue damage. When coupled with Alzheimer's drug administration, the technique could allow for much better pharmacological success rates, since the major cause of current drug trial failures are due to the blood-brain barrier preventing the drug from accessing the brain. Another fascinating line of research has resulted in the engineering of a nanodevice that can easily cross the blood-brain barrier. Once it enters the brain, it removes beta-amyloid peptides before they accumulate and form the sticky plaques known to cause downstream havoc in Alzheimer's disease. As Dr. Elena Rozhkova, one of the scientists involved with the project has phrased it, "the idea is that, eventually, a slurry of our nanodevices could collect the peptides as they fall away from the cells—before they get a chance to aggregate. We've . . . engineer[ed] a high-capacity 'cage' that traps the peptides and clears them from the brain." The same researchers tested the nanodevice in the brains of mice with Alzheimer's disease and found that they demonstrated the ability to reduce plaques by 30%, which could translate to a slower progression of disease.

The research presented in this chapter provides several exciting glimpses of what may be available for Alzheimer's disease patients in the coming years or decades. However, it will take some time for many of these new developments to reach the public (provided that they do not fizzle out first, as they move through more rigorous clinical trials). For good reason, many studies are needed to support the effectiveness of any particular medical advancement, and a robust safety profile must be observed before these technologies can be offered to the people who need them most. However, great strides have been made over the past several years, and the expanding knowledge base about the importance of preclinical assessment and treatment may herald a new era in Alzheimer's disease management.

Case Illustrations

JANE: EARLY DIAGNOSIS

Jane, a former schoolteacher, is 73 years old. She lives with her husband, William, who encouraged her to make an appointment with her physician. William has been concerned because Jane just hasn't seemed like her usual self lately. Recently, Jane has been frustrating her family by repeatedly asking them questions they have already answered. She is forgetting parts of conversations that they had only moments ago, and this prompted William to start seeking more answers. Her husband came with her to the office consultation and brought notes on what he thought would be helpful for the doctor to know. William initially did not want to consider that his wife might be developing dementia, but the possibility keeps crossing his mind, especially because they had taken care of her mother, who had suffered from Alzheimer's disease many years ago.

Jane and her husband went to her primary care physician's office to inquire about her new lapses in memory. She was nervous going in and downplayed some of her symptoms. The physician began by interviewing the Jane and her spouse in order to obtain a detailed history of her "presenting problem." In other words, the doctor asked questions about the symptoms that led her to make an appointment and whether any of Jane's biological relatives had ever experienced similar problems with thinking or memory. This was followed by a physical examination. The physician observed Jane from the moment he walked into the exam room. He looked for any immediate physical signs that would help him formulate a diagnosis, such as whether she was dressed appropriately for the weather and whether she maintained appropriate hygiene. These observations sometimes allow physicians to evaluate the severity of a person's mental decline. He also observed Jane throughout their interaction for any other noticeable signs such as defensiveness during questioning, engagement in the conversation, and coherence of her speech. Vital signs were measured to get a baseline for the health of essential organ systems that support the brain. Weight was also checked, as an unintentional weight loss in an older person is concerning and warrants further medical evaluation.

The physician conducted a neurologic exam next to assess the functioning of Jane's nervous system. This consisted of a sensory exam to test some of her cranial nerves and to check for sensory impairment. A gait test was also performed to observe her motor functions; the physician asked Jane to stand and walk around the room while he observed her movement and posture. The doctor also conducted the Mini-Mental State Exam (MMSE) during this part of the visit. Here he assessed her short-term memory, attention, and some other facets of thinking by asking her questions such as the current date and to perform tasks such as counting backward from 100 by sequential sevens (e.g., 100, 93, 86, etc.) At the end of the visit, he ordered blood tests to check blood cell counts to see whether the body was fighting infection and whether the kidneys and liver were properly functioning. After assessing her symptoms, Jane's physician provided a referral to a neurologist so that brain scan images could be collected, which could further clarify the origin of Jane's cognitive deficits. The neurologist opted for a computerized tomography (CT) scan instead of a magnetic resonance imaging (MRI) assessment, because Jane appeared distressed at the thought of being tightly enclosed within a loud machine. After the scans were completed, the neurologist looked for shrinkage of the brain as well as signs of bleeding or tumors. Jane was also referred to a neuropsychologist so that additional cognitive testing could be completed. A battery of cognitive tests was provided to further evaluate the mental deficits that were initially observed in the MMSE screening. Psychometric test results indicated that Jane experienced the most problems with language-based skills and in recalling items from short- and long-term memory. This crucial part of the evaluation took a few hours to complete and left Jane feeling mentally fatigued but also hopeful that the full extent of her condition could be better understood. After the neurological and neuropsychological testing were completed, Jane's primary doctor consulted with the other assessment providers and scheduled a follow-up appointment with Jane to discuss the overall test findings and conclusions. A probable diagnosis of early-stage Alzheimer's disease was made on the basis of Jane's observed impairments and the ruling out of other potential diagnoses that could have otherwise accounted for her decline in language and memory skills.

Analysis

One of the main concerns during the diagnostic stage is ruling out any diagnoses that may account for the presenting symptoms. A full health assessment is conducted that helps the physician discern what is going on inside the patient's body. Here the physician took note of family history that put the patient at increased risk for Alzheimer's disease. Current levels of physical, mental, and social impairment were assessed through various tests. This helped establish a baseline and monitor future progression of the disease. Correct diagnosis is essential for developing a targeted treatment plan to assist the individual through the progression of the illness.

The diagnosis of Alzheimer's disease is not one that anyone wants to receive. Its progressive nature and eventual terminal nature are frightening, and the gradual loss of independence and change in identity feel like they take away one's dignity. There is currently no cure for the disease, but identifiable risks can be minimized through consistent care for one's overall health. Physical, mental, and social health are all important to maintain. A balanced, low-carbohydrate diet and regular exercise have been shown to decrease chances of developing Alzheimer's disease, as does maintaining good sleep habits. Staying mentally active by trying new things and challenging the mind helps the brain stay fit. Social interactions are important for emotional health and help encourage more physical activity as well as stimulating the mind through conversation. All types of health are interconnected, and continued care and maintenance of what we have control over can help mitigate the fear of risk factors that are out of our control, such as age and genetic predisposition to disease.

ROGER: MILD ALZHEIMER'S DISEASE

Roger is a 76-year-old retired mechanic with early-stage Alzheimer's disease. He was diagnosed two years ago, after his wife finally convinced him to receive an evaluation. The couple lives together in the town where he used to work at a repair shop, and he still fills in for the occasional shift when someone calls off. Their three daughters often visit with their grandchildren. He argues a lot more with his family than he did before the memory decline started, because he does not acknowledge some of the changes his family members have pointed out.

Roger has been losing things, such as his keys, more often for the past few years, but he worried his wife recently when he lost his wedding ring for a week. He took it off before going into work at the repair shop as he always did, since the metal band is a safety hazard there, but he could not remember where he left it this time. He was embarrassed at first and then became upset with himself when he finally did find it when looking for something else in his dresser.

His wife reports that some of his old friends from the shop have also noticed changes in Roger's behavior. When filling in shifts, he often meets a lot of new people. He was always good at remembering names but seems to struggle with learning the names of new customers and employees. He seemed confused when one of his old work buddies thanked him for filling in for him the previous day. Roger completely forgot that he had been to the shop the day before. His daughter became worried when she got a flat tire and called her father to help her out. He seemed slow and unsure about the steps necessary to complete the job. She had seen him do it several times before with well-practiced speed, but this time he needed to restart a couple of times. At one point, he put the wrench down and stared at the tire blankly for a moment before shaking his head and trying again. He snapped when she asked if he needed help, and her feelings were hurt by his uncharacteristic moodiness.

His wife became concerned when his grandson asked if "Grandpappy was okay" after the two came home from the park on one Sunday afternoon. Her grandson told her that Roger yelled at him when the two were in the toolshed earlier that morning. Roger could not come up with the name of a tool he had lost the day before and tried to get his grandson to help him locate it after describing its size and shape. The search was unsuccessful. A short while later, Roger once again became upset and blamed his grandson for misplacing a different tool that the boy swore he did not touch. Roger was usually patient and kind, so his grandson initially thought that Roger must have been in a bad mood, maybe because he got up too early that morning. However, the boy started to think that something was wrong later that afternoon when the two got lost when walking back home from a local ice cream shop. Roger has lived in the same area for decades and had walked to the ice cream shop dozens of times before, but he seemed confused and disoriented at each street intersection. Because the trip home took nearly an hour longer than usual, his grandson got scared when he thought they were going to stay lost. Roger refused to call for directions, and they returned home late for dinner.

Roger at first repeatedly told his doctor that there were no changes going on with him and that his wife was "just hysterical." One thing he did admit to was missing lasagna. It had been his favorite food for years, but he was getting frustrated with his increased difficulty in using eating utensils and had started opting for finger foods in public to avoid embarrassment. With a little more prompting from the doctor, Roger also admitted to hiding some of his forgetfulness by keeping a little notebook with him, where he started writing down reminders for appointments and other things he needed to do. He missed his dental appointment the previous month and kept forgetting some of the groceries his wife wanted him to pick up. He never liked asking anyone for help and said he did not want anyone to think that he could not take care of his family.

Analysis

It is not uncommon for patients to be reluctant or even vocally resistant to coming in for an evaluation. Even when familiar with their doctor and having an established relationship built on trust, the aging process is scary. The words *dementia* or *Alzheimer's disease* are even more so. Often, patients at this stage do not see some of the changes that are occurring within them. This can lead to arguments with family, which can be exacerbated by the mood changes that start to occur from the disease.

In this case, the patient started noticing some symptoms and was trying to hide them. This is also common. As daily functioning becomes more impaired, reflected in difficulties with eating and hygiene, the condition becomes harder to hide and more difficult to manage. At this stage, his family was okay with him driving. In time, increased confusion, loss of motor control, and impaired judgment that will follow with the progression of the disease will cause him to lose his privilege to drive. He was also able to pick up occasional shifts at work. As his memory continues to decline and he loses other functions, this will soon not be possible for him. Changes brought about by the disease at the early stage are particularly hard on the individual, because the desire to continue life as it was is prominent, and awareness that something is off is frustrating.

KIRK: MODERATE ALZHEIMER'S DISEASE

Kirk is currently 81 years old, and he was diagnosed with Alzheimer's disease five years ago. He is a retired music instructor, and his wife passed away 15 years ago. They did not have any children together. His nephew, who helped him run his music school, is now his primary caregiver. His nephew reported that Kirk's memory problems started in his late 60s, but the symptoms were not severe enough at the time for him to see them as anything but normal aging. Kirk's wife was still alive at that time and was his primary social contact. His early personality changes and worsening forgetfulness were attributed to her death. He is currently experiencing the middle stages of Alzheimer's disease.

The progression of the disease has been hard on his nephew, as it seems his uncle is becoming a different person. Notably, the once-devoted cello player has not picked up his instrument in six months. Kirk remembered that he needed to do something with the bow, but he could not remember the steps to tighten and rosin it. After putting the bow down in frustration, he did not remember the incident when his nephew asked him about it 20 minutes later. Kirk also snaps at his caregiver frequently over little things that did not bother him before. His nephew tries not to take things personally, but he called the doctor's office very concerned when his uncle accused him of stealing. The patient could not find his wallet, and they searched the house up and down for three days before finding it in the freezer. The same day it was found, Kirk did not remember accusing his nephew.

The patient's memory is noticeably changing. Kirk did not recognize his nephew's best friend, whom he has known for 30 years. He became confused when the friend came by to stay with the patient so Kirk's nephew could run errands. The interaction upset Kirk because he was frustrated that he could not remember who this person was. As a man of a generation encouraged to hide feelings, Kirk surprised his nephew and his friend when he became tearful over the encounter. The caregiver reported that the patient's mood changes are becoming more frequent and unpredictable.

Once a proud man with regard to appearance, Kirk now expresses frustration with his nephew when it comes to hygiene. He seems confused about what is being asked when his caregiver prompts that it is time to take a shower. He needs some help with dressing, as buttons and other fastenings can be too difficult. He does not seem bothered to be in the same wrinkled clothing for a couple days at a time, while others fight with him to get clean.

His nephew still tries to maintain as much of their old routine as he can while adapting for the extra time it takes to get ready and the changes in his uncle's functioning. At church, Kirk started laughing loudly in the middle of the pastor's sermon. He seemed confused as to why his nephew asked him to lower his voice, and they left mass early when Kirk would not calm down. He got particularly agitated on their way out, because he got lost looking for the bathroom when his nephew said to wait inside while he pulled up the car. His nephew was scared when he did not see his uncle waiting at the door as instructed and was concerned when he found Kirk. His uncle had wandered downstairs looking for the bathroom even though they have attended this church for over 20 years and the bathrooms were on the main level.

Analysis

The patient requires increased care as the disease progresses, but his caregiver tries to keep him mentally active by doing puzzles with him and reading Bible verses with him. Kirk has decreased mobility, but they do tend a tomato garden together in the yard when the weather is good and go for walks on days when he has more energy.

It is important for clinicians to rule out other potential diagnoses, such as depression, but it is difficult sometimes to correctly differentiate symptoms. The presence of either dementia or depression also does not rule out the possibility of having the other. Kirk's primary care physician had treated him and his wife for decades, and it was unfortunate that the complication of the patient's wife passing muddied his assessment of symptoms early on. Changes in the brain often occur before a patient is diagnosed, as it takes time for the effects on the brain to be compounded enough to produce noticeable changes in memory and behavior. Kirk's nephew was shocked and scared at how quickly his uncle's memory had worsened and his personality seemed to change recently. The longer a patient goes without diagnosis, the quicker the decline can seem to occur to family, when the disease has, in fact, been ravaging the brain for years.

Although the early stages of Alzheimer's disease are marked by impairments to short-term memory, the middle stages are typically characterized by a decline in long-term memory. The effects of forgetting things such as birthdays and names can be hurtful to family members, and individuals who are trying to recall this type of information are often left feeling frustrated by their inability to remember things that were once easily retrievable. This difficulty, which is often easier for the patient to ignore in earlier stages, is further compounded by personality changes that are typical of the moderate Alzheimer's stage. Caregivers often mention that their loved ones do not report feeling like their old selves, and they regularly observe uncharacteristic behaviors, verbalizations, and mood states when the patient reaches the middle stage of the disease.

Unfortunately, there is no cure for Alzheimer's disease. Management of the disease is done through pharmacological or nonpharmacological means. Pharmacological interventions are often not the initial treatment, and when they are used, they are often recommended in conjunction with lifestyle changes. The patient in this case has increased dependence on his caregiver, and, at the doctor's recommendation, there are continued efforts to initiate mental, physical, and social stimulation to help slow the decline. Right now, Kirk is able to live at home and has his nephew to care for him. His nephew is able to occasionally step out for brief errands. As the disease progresses, management will require full-time care that may exhaust his nephew to the point where they need outside help or even the placement of Kirk in a care facility.

ETHEL: SEVERE ALZHEIMER'S DISEASE

Ethel is an 84-year-old patient who was diagnosed with severe Alzheimer's disease seven years ago and is currently in the final stage of the disease. Five months ago, she had a concerning increase in hospital visits, and her doctors recommended a change in care to her family. Her full-time support was encouraged to shift from a focus on stimulation (formerly in place to attempt to slow her decline) to a focus on comfort measures to ease her through the end stage of her life. It was a hard decision to make, but she was moved from the nursing home to a hospice care facility. As a former secretary, it was particularly difficult for her family to watch her once lively personality recede as the illness progressed. Ethel had a friendly personality and was never afraid to meet or talk to new people. She grew up as a Polish American immigrant and used to love telling stories about her childhood to anyone who would listen. A couple months ago, her speech became limited to around five words per day, and the only words that did come out were in her native tongue. A Polish nun that visits her daily for prayer and to read her the Bible says that the few words Ethel used to say did not make sense. Recently, she stopped talking altogether.

Several weeks back, other daily activities became increasingly difficult for Ethel or impossible for her to do on her own. Staff at the facility are very careful during her mealtimes, as she is more prone to choking than she was before because she now has difficulty swallowing. She has to be reminded to chew food when it is in her mouth and would let it sit in her cheeks if she went unprompted. Her family was saddened to see her weight loss and that drinking is also a chore for her now. Years ago, she used to pride herself on the coffee she made for her family every morning, but now she is limited in what she is served to drink. Ethel is unable to sit up without assistance and needs to be shifted by the staff at her facility. She used to love going for daily walks. After she became immobile, the staff used to take her for regular afternoon walks in a wheelchair. They still change her position in her room to help minimize the chance of developing bedsores and try to get her natural sunlight from the windows during the day, but it is too much stress on her body to move her a lot. It was very hard for Ethel's daughter to learn that her mother suffers from incontinence. Ethel was always an old-fashioned woman who valued privacy, and her daughter became tearful when learning of this development. The staff assured her they are very careful to preserve Ethel's dignity, but some changes to a patient's life are a lot for family to have to hear and see.

Ethel's doctors feel she does not have much time left and are glad that her family was able to plan ahead for these final moments because the diagnosis was given years ago. One of her family members is at the facility as often as is allowed to watch for signs of discomfort and distress. They want to be as supportive as they can during Ethel's last days, but they are not sure how to do so, because Ethel often does not recognize her family. The staff is apologetic when they ask the family to leave the room at times because she gets upset at "new" faces. Staff report that she spends most of her time sleeping and drifting into unconsciousness, but she is restless at almost all times when awake. At the nursing home and in her first days at the hospice facility, she had more predictable periods of agitation as evening came on and throughout the night. Her daughter reports it is difficult to see her mother swing from so sedated and with shallow breathing at rest to wide-eyed when awake. She still holds Ethel's hand when her mother is resting, but it makes her sad to notice that her skin is now cold to the touch. Ethel's daughter finds comfort in the fact that her mother no longer remembers some of her most painful memories. For example, Ethel has forgotten that she lost her husband and son in a drunk driving accident 15 years ago. Her daughter hopes Ethel's final moment is completely free of mental and physical pain.

Analysis

As we have seen, there is no cure for Alzheimer's disease. At best, the medications on the market slow down the disease, but they do not stop or reverse its effects. The most common treatment plan involves a combination of medication and alternative treatments. This disease requires treating the whole person, with a focus on trying to slow the course of the disease in its early stages and maintaining the patient's dignity in its later stages.

The patient is to be kept as physically, mentally, and socially active as possible for as long as can be. It is important to keep the person physically well by providing a balanced diet with food that can be easily swallowed without risk of choking. Light physical activities such as walking are encouraged to keep the body mobile and strong until the disease removes this option. The patient should also be socially engaged when able. As the disease progresses, it may be through routine conversations with the caregiver while still in the comfort of the home. In all of these domains, it is important to note that routines should not be disrupted and too many new people and unfamiliar places should not be introduced, as this may do more harm than good by startling and confusing the individual. This can be hurtful for the patient's family, as observed in Ethel's case.

Alzheimer's disease has a different course in every individual and consequently requires unique treatment for every profile and adjustments as it progresses. The caregiver must be in tune with the patient and alert the medical staff of any significant changes to the patient. Losing independence takes away part of someone's identity, and losing control of basic functions such as control over bowel and bladder movements is not the way anyone intends for their later years to be spent. Changes of living situation, such as moving to a nursing home, is understandably scary for someone who is already disoriented in once familiar places. Decisions for the family, such as when to move to more advanced care plans, are incredibly difficult to make, and planning is best done early, as seen here.

NANCY: AN INFORMAL FAMILY CAREGIVER

Nancy is 57 and takes care of mother Helen, 79, who has been diagnosed with Alzheimer's disease. Helen's husband, Ken, was her primary caregiver early on, but he passed away three years ago from a heart attack. Nancy had to take on his role, and it was manageable with her work schedule at first. Helen required far less care in the beginning: Nancy was able to work full time and pop in for a daily visit. Early on, she would make sure her mother was keeping appointments, help her stay on track with bills, and check to see if she remembered to take her medication. She would help with planning grocery lists and see to it that her mother's house was fully stocked with food and other essentials. After Helen started missing doctor's appointments, it was clear that she needed more than a quick check-in. Nancy started to become responsible for scheduling doctor visits to keep tabs on the course of the disease and to monitor her mother's existing health issues of type 2 diabetes and hypertension. Helen used to prepare her own notes for doctor's visits, but now Nancy writes down her mother's questions, tracks medication and changes in symptoms, and tries to plan ahead to arrive early and make the appointments less stressful for Helen. Nancy used to take Helen out for lunch after her medical appointments, but as time went by, visits to medical professionals started to leave Helen feeling fatigued and mentally depleted, so now they usually enjoy lunch and a quiet afternoon at home afterward. At appointments, Nancy takes notes to remember things later and frequently asks questions about the next stages, to plan ahead.

Nancy has mixed feelings about her role as a caregiver. At first, she was grateful to be able to give back to the woman who raised her. But at the same time, the position has never been easy. Watching her mother's mental and physical health decline has been terrifying for Nancy, and the demands of caretaking have become increasingly demanding over the past several months. Nancy feels guilty for experiencing moments of resentment toward Helen. She knows that Alzheimer's disease is the reason why her mother swears and hits her when it is time to take medication. But these extreme personality changes make it difficult for Nancy to remain understanding at all times.

Some days, she feels helpless and at a loss for what to do for her mother. Nancy calls the doctor for advice, sometimes late at night when there is a new symptom or a worsening of a long-standing problem. She knew it would be a hard and long process, but the daily difficulties have compounded over time and made her frustrated by the situation for herself and her mother. Nancy has many sleepless nights because Helen is restless and needs more care, and there is little to no respite during the day because she is busy attending to the house and other necessary tasks, such as meal preparation and scheduling. Nancy started counseling six months ago to have a place to process her changing identity and talk about her complicated feelings. She has found the experience helpful and is learning to accept that it is human to get upset at her situation. At her counselor's recommendation, Nancy is going to start attending a local support group for caregivers a few times a week. Nancy is encouraged that there are people in her community who understand her circumstances but is a little nervous to talk to a group of people about her personal life. Helen's friend from church, Sue, comes over to let Nancy have time to go grocery shopping for the house and to run other errands, and Nancy's childhood best friend stops by a few times a week to watch Helen, so Nancy can schedule appointments and make other arrangements for her mother. Nancy is happy that Helen is able to see a few familiar faces and stay socially engaged for now. Previously, she used to drop off Helen at an adult day care center a few times a week so that Helen could be socially stimulated, which allowed Nancy to catch up on sleep and take care of herself. But unfortunately, the busy day care environment became too stressful for Helen, prompting Nancy to take over caregiving responsibilities in a full-time capacity.

Nancy loves her mother and wants to keep caring for her as long as possible, but she does get understandably stressed about the situation. Finances are difficult because Nancy is unmarried, and Helen's husband left the family with medical bills when he died. Nancy used to be able to work and take care of her mother, but the increased demands of the caregiver role required her to retire earlier than she ever expected. Nancy's former boss could not allow the frequent absences and short notices of taking time off. Nancy misses her former career and is not financially stable. She is stalling on sending her mother to a nursing home because she really wants to provide personal care as long as she can, and she simply cannot afford to place her mother in a round-the-clock assisted living facility.

Analysis

After a patient receives a diagnosis, the burden of the disease falls most heavily on the primary caregiver, who is often a family member. Caregivers typically feel exhausted emotionally, mentally, physically, and financially. Day-to-day difficulties and complications increase fatigue and deplete a caregiver's resources across all four of these areas. Watching loved ones deteriorate gradually and progressively lose personality traits, interests, and abilities that made those people who they were takes a large toll on the family. Even just a typical day of being a caregiver can be emotionally exhausting. Going through extreme moments of sadness at seeing a loved one in this state, feeling guilt or defeat at self-perceived inadequacies in providing care, and being hurt by personal verbal attacks from a loved one who does not really mean them is understandably draining.

Mentally, being a caregiver is a significant adjustment to cope with. A caregiver may start with only a few hours of monitoring or running errands for an individual at the start of the disease, but the nature of Alzheimer's disease requires more intensive care as the disease progresses. Personal responsibility for a loved one could cause someone to stay in and commit to a job that they never asked or planned for. Most caregivers are family members, and anytime someone with an existing relationship becomes a caregiver, an adjustment of roles occurs. The grandson who is still learning how to take care of himself must now step in and take care of someone else. The husband who did minimal housework must now take on his wife's duties. In Nancy's case, the daughter who was once cared for now must provide care to her mother. It is unfamiliar territory from the moment the role is stepped into, and it continues to change for the entire course of the disease as the patient's needs evolve.

The patient is not the only one to be physically damaged by the disease. A petite caregiver may injure herself trying to assist the larger patient in walking and maneuvering in the bathtub. Chronic sleep deprivation caused by monitoring the patient for nighttime wandering and assisting with frequent nighttime bathroom trips wrecks the caregiver's chance at recovering at night from exhaustion.

Perhaps the easiest thing to quantify is the financial burden on caregivers. In the United States, there are 16 million unpaid caregivers providing care to a loved one. Caregiving may result in lost time at work, temporarily quitting a job, or early retirement, as we saw with Nancy. The caregiver delivers better care when provided support. Interventions that initially improve caregiving competency, gradually address the care needs of the person living with dementia, and offer emotional support for loss and grief when needed tend to be most effective. Keep in mind, support for the caregiver should be adjusted as the role intensifies and becomes more demanding as the disease progresses.

Glossary

Acetylcholine (ACh)
A type of neurotransmitter that plays a critical role in memory and cognition.

Acetylcholinesterase (AChE)
An enzyme that catalyzes the breakdown of acetylcholine.

Activities of daily living (ADLs)
Fundamental skills that are required to independently care for oneself.

Age-related macular degeneration
An eye disease that results from damage to the part of the retina called the macula, which causes loss of central vision.

Allele
A form or variation of a gene.

Alzheimer's dementia
Used to describe people in the dementia stage of the continuum of Alzheimer's.

Alzheimer's disease
A degenerative brain disease that destroys memory and other important mental functions.

Amyloid beta
Peptides of amino acids that are the main component of the amyloid plaques found in the brains of people with Alzheimer's disease.

Amyloid hypothesis
The assumption that accumulation of $A\beta$ in the brain is the primary influence driving Alzheimer's disease pathogenesis.

Amyloid plaques
Aggregates of misfolded amyloid beta proteins that form in the spaces between nerve cells.

Amyloid precursor protein (APP)
A common membrane protein of unknown primary function that is found in many body tissues and concentrated in the synapses of neurons.

Antagonist (drug)
A type of drug that avoids or decreases a biological reaction.

Apathy
The lack of interest, enthusiasm, or concern.

APOE ε4
Gene variation that is a known risk factor for late-onset Alzheimer's disease.

Apolipoprotein E (APOE) gene
A gene on chromosome 19 involved in making a protein that helps carry cholesterol and other types of fat in the bloodstream. It comes in several different variations: APOE ε2, APOE ε3, and APOE ε4.

Autobiographical memory
Episodes recollected from an individual's life, based on a combination of episodic and semantic memory.

Baby boom generation
A generational cohort generally defined as people born from 1946 to 1964, during the post–World War II increase in birth rates.

Behavioral disturbances
Manifestations of underlying psychological disturbances that impair perception, behavior, or mood.

Beta-amyloid protein
Small piece of the larger amyloid precursor protein (APP).

Beta secretase
An enzyme that cleaves amyloid precursor protein, thereby assisting in the formation of amyloid beta.

Biomarker
A measurable substance in an organism whose presence is indicative of some phenomenon such as disease, infection, or environmental exposure.

Blood-brain barrier
A capillary network surrounding the brain made up of specialized cells that blocks large, non-lipid soluble molecules in the bloodstream from entering the brain.

Brain cell
(See Neuron.)

Brain-derived neurotropic factor (BDNF)
A key molecule involved in nerve cell growth and survival and in neuroplastic changes within the brain that relate to learning and memory.

Brain tissue
Tissue made up of neurons and glial cells.

Brain wave
A frequency of synchronized electrical pulses in the brain produced by masses of neurons communicating with each other.

Cardiovascular disease (CVD)
A disease of the heart or blood vessels.

Cataracts
A condition affecting the eye that causes clouding of the lens.

Cell receptor
Area on a receiving neuron that a neurotransmitter or drug molecule binds to in order to produce some type of cellular response.

Central nervous system
The part of the nervous system consisting primarily of the brain and spinal cord.

Cerebral cortex
A thin layer of neural tissue that covers the outermost portion (1.5 mm to 5 mm) of the brain.

Cerebrospinal fluid (CSF)
A clear, colorless body fluid found in the brain and spinal cord, produced by cells inside the brain.

Cerebrospinal fluid (CSF) assay
A series of laboratory tests performed on CSF, used to obtain biomarker evidence for the presence of Alzheimer's disease.

Ceruminous glands
Specialized sweat glands located subcutaneously in the external auditory canal.

Cholinesterase inhibitor
A group of medicines that block the normal breakdown of acetylcholine.

Chromosome
A compact structure containing DNA and proteins present in nearly all cells of the body.

Chronic traumatic encephalopathy (CTE)
A progressive brain disease associated with repeated brain trauma, including concussions and repeated blows to the head.

Chronology
The sequential order in which past events occur.

Clinical interview
A commonly used assessment procedure that involves a clinician asking questions in order to gather information needed for diagnosis and treatment.

Clinical significance (symptoms)
Quality of causing significant distress or impairment in social, occupational, or other important areas of functioning.

Clinical trials
Research studies performed in people that are aimed at evaluating a medical, surgical, or behavioral intervention.

C9ORF72
Gene that provides instructions for making a protein that is found in various tissues.

Cognitive rehabilitation
A class of nonpharmacological treatment for dementia that does not set out to train or improve cognition but uses a goal-oriented approach to facilitate the management of functional disability.

Cognitive reserve
Extent to which the brain can sustain damage before intellectual capacity is affected.

Cognitive reserve theory
Postulation that individual differences in the cognitive processes or neural networks underlying task performance allow some people to cope better than others with brain damage.

Cognitive stimulation
A range of activities (e.g., games, sensory exercises) and discussions (e.g., talking about past experiences) usually carried out in small groups of three to six patients, with the aim of general enhancement of cognitive and social functioning.

Cognitive training
A class of nonpharmacological treatment for dementia that focuses on guided practice on tasks that target specific cognitive functions, such as memory, attention, or problem-solving.

Complication
An unanticipated problem that arises following, and is a result of, a procedure, treatment, or illness.

Computed tomography (CT/CAT)
A noninvasive diagnostic-imaging procedure that uses special X-ray measurements to produce axial images (often called "slices") of the brain.

Control group
The group in an experiment or study that does not receive treatment by the researchers and is used as a benchmark to measure how the other tested subjects perform.

Coronary artery disease
A condition where the major blood vessels become narrowed and cannot supply enough oxygen-rich blood to the heart.

Correlation
The degree to which variables are related.

Correlational study
A type of research design where a researcher seeks to understand whether naturally occurring variables are related.

Cortical thickness
A brain measure used to describe the combined thickness of the layers of the cerebral cortex in mammalian brains, either in local terms or as a global average for the entire brain.

Crystallized intelligence
Knowledge people acquire through life experience and education.

CT/CAT (computed tomography) scan
Procedure using several X-ray images and computer processing to create cross-sectional images of a person's body.

Cystic fibrosis
A genetic disorder that affects the way the body makes mucus that makes it difficult to breathe and can cause lung damage.

Delirium
A temporary mental state characterized by confusion, anxiety, incoherent speech, and hallucinations.

Delusion
An idiosyncratic belief or impression that is firmly maintained despite being contradicted by what is generally accepted as reality or rational argument and that is typically a symptom of mental disorder.

Dementia
A general term for loss of memory, language, and problem-solving and other thinking abilities that is severe enough to interfere with daily life; Alzheimer's disease is the most common form.

Deoxyribonucleic acid (DNA)
The hereditary material in humans and almost all other organisms.

Diabetes, type 1
A long-term, autoimmune condition in which the pancreas produces little or no insulin, thereby preventing blood sugar from entering into cells and causing it to build up in the bloodstream.

Diabetes, type 2
A long-term condition in which the pancreas produces insulin, but the body does not effectively respond to it, thereby preventing blood sugar from entering into cells and causing it to build up in the bloodstream.

Diagnostic and Statistical Manual of Mental Disorders (*DSM*-5)
The handbook used by health-care professionals in the United States and much of the world as the authoritative guide to the diagnosis of mental disorders; contains descriptions, symptoms, and other criteria for diagnosing mental disorders.

Diagnostic criteria
Specific signs, symptoms, and other requirements that must be met by the patient before a formal diagnosis is made.

Differential diagnosis
A process wherein a clinician differentiates between two or more conditions that could be behind a person's symptoms.

Disorientation
The inability to correctly acknowledge the current time, place, one's role, and personal identity.

Donepezil
A medication prescribed to treat symptoms of mild to moderate and moderate to severe Alzheimer's disease, sold as the trade name Aricept, which works by preventing the breakdown of acetylcholine in the brain.

Dorsomedial prefrontal cortex
An area in the prefrontal cortex of the brain involved in various functions, such as attention, emotion, and decision-making.

Double-blind study
A type of research investigation in which neither the participants nor the experimenters know who is receiving a particular treatment.

Early-onset Alzheimer's disease (EOAD)
Alzheimer's disease diagnosed before the age of 65.

Effectiveness
The performance of an intervention under "real-world" conditions.

Efficacy
The performance of an intervention under ideal and controlled circumstances.

Entorhinal cortex
Small structure embedded in the anterior temporal lobe involved in memory.

Enzyme-linked immunosorbent assay (ELISA)
A plate-based assay technique designed for detecting and quantifying soluble substances such as peptides, proteins, antibodies, and hormones.

Episodic memory
Recollection of personal experiences and specific objects, people, and events experienced at a particular time and place.

Etiology
The origin of a disease.

Familial Alzheimer's disease (FAD)
When two or more people in a family are diagnosed with Alzheimer's disease.

Fibril
A small fiber.

Food and Drug Administration (FDA)
A federal agency of the Department of Health and Human Services that is responsible for protecting the public health by ensuring the safety, efficacy, and security of human and veterinary drugs, biological products, the national food supply, and other consumable products.

Frontotemporal degeneration (FTD)
A group of brain disorders caused by degeneration of the frontal and/or temporal lobes of the brain.

Functional brain imaging
A process used to identify brain areas and underlying brain processes that are associated with performing a particular cognitive or behavioral task.

Functional magnetic resonance imaging (fMRI)
A functional brain-imaging method that measures brain activity by detecting changes associated with blood flow.

Galantamine
A medication prescribed to treat symptoms of mild to moderate Alzheimer's disease, sold under the brand name Razadyne, which works by preventing the breakdown of acetylcholine and stimulating the brain to release more acetylcholine.

Gamma secretase
An enzyme that cleaves amyloid precursor protein, thereby assisting in the formation of amyloid beta.

Gamma wave
A 30 Hz to 100 Hz brain wave that decreases in the brains of Alzheimer's disease patients; It is associated with higher-order brain functions.

Gene
A basic unit of heredity. Genes direct a cell to make proteins and guide almost every aspect of a cell's construction, operation, and repair.

Genetic mutation
A permanent alteration in the DNA sequence that makes up a gene such that the sequence differs from what is found in most people.

Genetic variant
One of two or more alternative forms of a gene that arise by mutation and are found at the same place on a chromosome (also called an allele).

Genotyping
The process of determining differences in the genetic makeup (genotype) of an individual by examining the individual's DNA sequence.

Glaucoma
A condition of increased pressure within the eye, causing gradual loss of sight if left untreated.

Glutamate
The most abundant excitatory neurotransmitter in the vertebrate nervous system.

Glymphatic system
A network of vessels that clear waste from the central nervous system (CNS), mostly during sleep.

Hallucination
An experience involving the apparent perception of something not present.

Hippocampus
A brain structure that is involved in the formation of new memories and is also associated with learning and emotions.

Hormone
A regulatory substance produced in an organism and transported in tissue fluids, such as blood or sap, to stimulate specific cells or tissues into action.

Hydrocephalus
An abnormal accumulation of cerebrospinal fluid (CSF) within the cavities of the brain.

Hyperglycemia
High levels of sugar, or glucose, in the blood, which occurs when the body does not produce or use enough insulin.

Hypertension
Abnormally high blood pressure.

Inflammation
The complex biological response of body tissues to harmful stimuli, such as pathogens, damaged cells, or irritants, that is a protective response involving immune cells and blood vessels.

Informal caretaker
Someone who provides care services, typically unpaid, to someone with whom the individual has a personal relationship.

Insomnia
Difficulty initiating or maintaining sleep.

Instrumental activities of daily living (IADLs)
Tasks necessary for independent living that do not necessarily have to be done every single day.

Insulin
A hormone produced in the pancreas that regulates the amount of glucose in the blood.

Insulin resistance
A condition in which the body's cells become resistant to the effects of insulin, resulting in the need for higher levels of insulin in order for insulin to have its proper effects.

***International Classification of Diseases* (ICD-10)**
A globally used diagnostic tool for epidemiology, health management, and clinical purposes, maintained by the World Health Organization (WHO).

Ketogenic diet
A low-carb, high-fat diet. It lowers blood sugar and insulin levels and shifts the body's metabolism away from carbs and toward using fat for energy.

Ketosis
A metabolic state characterized by elevated levels of ketone bodies in the blood or urine.

Late-onset Alzheimer's disease (LOAD)
Alzheimer's disease diagnosed after the age of 65.

Lewy body dementia
A disease associated with abnormal deposits of proteins, called Lewy bodies, affecting chemicals in the brain and potentially leading to problems with thinking, movement, behavior, and mood.

Longitudinal study
A research design that involves repeated observations of the same individuals over a period of time.

Magnetic resonance imaging (MRI)
A medical imaging technique that uses a magnetic field and computer-generated radio waves to create detailed images of the human body.

Major depressive disorder
A psychological disorder characterized by a persistent feeling of sadness or a lack of interest in outside stimuli.

Major neurocognitive disorder
An acquired disorder of cognitive function that is commonly characterized by impairments in memory, speech, reasoning, intellectual function, and/or spatial-temporal awareness.

Medicaid
A federal and state program that helps with medical costs for some people with limited income and resources.

Medicare
The official U.S. health insurance program for people age 65 or older.

Medium-chain triglycerides (MCTs)
Fats that come from coconut oil, palm oil, and butter.

Memantine
A medication prescribed to treat symptoms of moderate to severe Alzheimer's disease, sold under the brand name Namenda, which works by blocking the toxic effects associated with access glutamate.

Mental-status exam
The psychological equivalent of a physical exam that describes the mental state and behaviors of the person being seen.

Meta-analysis
A quantitative study design used to systematically assess the results of previous research to derive conclusions about that body of research.

Microglia
A neuronal support cell found in the central nervous system that functions primarily as an immune cell.

Microtubule
A microscopic tubular structure that gives structure and shape to a cell.

Mild cognitive impairment (MCI)
The stage between the expected cognitive decline of normal aging and the more serious decline of dementia that is characterized by problems with memory, language, thinking, or judgment. (See mild neurocognitive decline and prodromal dementia.)

Mild neurocognitive decline
The stage between the expected cognitive decline of normal aging and the more serious decline of dementia that is characterized by problems with memory, language, thinking, or judgment. (See mild cognitive impairment and prodromal dementia.)

Mindfulness
A mental state achieved by focusing one's awareness on the present moment, while calmly acknowledging and accepting one's feelings, thoughts, and bodily sensations.

Mindfulness-based stress reduction (MBSR)
A stress-reduction program that offers secular, intensive mindfulness training to assist people with stress, anxiety, depression, and pain.

Mini-Mental State Exam (MMSE)
A widely used test of cognitive function among the elderly; it includes tests of orientation, attention, memory, and language.

Mitochondria
Rod-shaped organelles that can be considered the power generators of a cell, converting oxygen and nutrients into energy.

Montreal Cognitive Assessment (MoCA)
A brief 30-question test that takes around 10 to 12 minutes to complete and helps assess people for dementia.

Motor control
The regulation of movement by the nervous system.

Mozart effect
The popular but incorrect assumption that listening to classical music can enhance the intelligence of people in general and babies in particular.

Music therapy
An evidence-based clinical use of musical interventions to improve clients' quality of life.

Nerve cell
(See neuron.)

Neurocognitive
Describes cognitive functions associated with specific pathways or loci within the brain that are affected by different disease processes.

Neurodegenerative disease
A disease that involves a progressive destruction of nerve cells.

Neurofibril
A fibril in the cytoplasm of a nerve cell, visible by light microscopy.

Neurofibrillary tangles
Abnormal accumulations of a protein called tau that collect inside neurons; they are commonly known as a primary marker of Alzheimer's disease.

Neurogenesis
The process by which new neurons are formed in the brain.

Neuroimaging
A class of technology that provides an array of visual representations of the structural anatomy of the nervous system.

Neurological assessment
A medical examination that assesses mental status, cranial nerves, motor and sensory function, pupillary response, reflexes, the cerebellum, and vital signs.

Neuron
A specialized cell designed to transmit information to other nerve, muscle, or gland cells, also called a brain cell or a nerve cell.

Neuropathology
Branch of medicine concerned with diseases of the nervous system.

Neuroplasticity
The ability of neural networks in the brain to change through growth and reorganization.

Neuroprotection
The preservation of neuronal structure and/or function.

Neuropsychological assessment
An evaluation to determine the extent of impairment to a particular ability and to attempt to determine the area of the brain that may have been damaged following brain injury or neurological illness.

Neurosyphilis
Refers to infection of the central nervous system in a patient with syphilis.

Neurotransmitter
A chemical message released by nerve cells to send signals to other cells, such as neurons, muscle cells, and gland cells.

Nonverbal memory
The ability to code, store, and recover information about faces, shapes, images, songs, sounds, smells, tastes, and feelings.

Nucleus basalis
An area near the center of the brain that contains many neurons that produce acetylcholine.

Optical coherence tomography (OCT)
A noninvasive, nondestructive means of 3D mapping the shape of the retina and optic nerve.

Optic nerve
A nerve that transmits visual information from the retina to the brain.

Parkinson's disease
A brain disorder that leads to shaking, stiffness, and difficulty with walking, balance, and coordination.

Pathophysiology
The disordered physiological processes associated with disease or injury.

Peptide
A compound consisting of two or more amino acids linked in a chain.

Perceptual-motor ability
The ability to interact with the environment by combining the use of one's senses and motor skills.

Physical examination
The examination of a patient for any possible medical signs or symptoms of a medical condition.

Placebo
A harmless pill, medicine, or procedure prescribed more for the psychological benefit of the patient than for any physiological effect.

Plasticity
The ability of neural networks in the brain to change through growth and reorganization.

Positron emission tomography (PET)
A functional imaging technique that uses radioactive substances known as radio-tracers to visualize and measure changes in metabolic processes and in other physiological activities such as blood flow, regional chemical composition, and absorption.

Preclinical Alzheimer's disease
The presence of Alzheimer's disease brain pathology without evidence of cognitive impairment; usually only diagnosed in research contexts.

Presbyopia
Farsightedness caused by loss of elasticity of the lens of the eye, occurring typically in middle and old age.

Presenile dementia
The onset of dementia before the age of 65.

Presenilin
Any of several proteins of cell membranes that are believed to contribute to the development of Alzheimer's disease.

Processing speed
A measure of the time required to respond to and/or process information in one's environment.

Prodromal dementia
The stage between the expected cognitive decline of normal aging and the more serious decline of dementia that is characterized by problems with memory, language, thinking, or judgment. (See mild cognitive impairment and mild neurocognitive decline.)

Prognosis
The likely course of a disease or ailment.

Protein
A substance that determines the physical and chemical characteristics of a cell and therefore of an organism. Proteins are essential to all cell functions and are created using genetic information.

Psychoanalysis
Psychological theory and therapy that aim to treat mental disorders by investigating the interaction of conscious and unconscious elements in the mind and bringing repressed fears and conflicts into the conscious mind by techniques such as dream interpretation and free association.

Psychomotor fatigue
A slowing-down of thought and a reduction of physical movements in an individual.

Psychosocial intervention
Interpersonal or informational activities, techniques, or strategies that target biological, behavioral, cognitive, emotional, interpersonal, social, or environmental factors with the aim of improving health functioning and well-being.

Psychotropic
Any drug that affects behavior, mood, thoughts, or perception.

Randomized controlled trial
A study design that randomly assigns participants into an experimental group or a control group.

Reality orientation
A program designed to improve cognitive and psychomotor function in persons who are confused or disoriented.

Retinal ganglion cell
A type of neuron located near the inner surface of the retina of the eye.

Rivastigmine
A medication prescribed to treat symptoms of mild to moderate Alzheimer's disease, sold under the brand name Exelon, which works by preventing the breakdown of acetylcholine and butyrylcholine.

Self-esteem
One's subjective evaluation of one's own worth.

Semantic memory
General knowledge and facts about the world.

Senile dementia
A term that was used for many years to describe older individuals who suffered from cognitive decline, particularly memory loss.

Senile plaque
A microscopic mass of fragmented and decaying nerve terminals around an amyloid core.

Serotonin
A neurotransmitter involved with a variety of functions, including modulating mood, cognition, reward, learning, memory, and numerous physiological processes.

Severe impairment battery
A series of tests used to assess cognition in patients with severe neurocognitive impairment.

Sickle cell anemia
An inherited blood disorder in which a mutated form of hemoglobin distorts the red blood cells into a crescent shape at low oxygen levels.

Side effects
Unwanted symptoms caused by a medical treatment.

Single-photon emission computed tomography (SPECT)
A noninvasive functional nuclear imaging test that shows how blood flows to tissues and organs.

Social cognition
A broad term used to describe cognitive processes related to the perception, understanding, and implementation of linguistic, auditory, visual, and physical cues that communicate emotional and interpersonal information.

Stroke
A sudden interruption in the blood supply of the brain.

Structural brain imaging
Approaches that are specialized for the visualization and analysis of anatomical properties of the brain.

Synapse
The site of transmission of electrochemical nerve impulses between two neurons.

Syphilis
A bacterial infection usually spread by sexual contact that starts as a painless sore typically on the genitals, rectum, or mouth.

Tau
A protein that helps stabilize the internal structure of nerve cells (microtubules).

Transcranial electromagnetic treatment (TEMT)
An electromagnetic field that penetrates brain cells in order to break up aggregated amyloid-beta and tau protein.

Translocase of outer mitochondrial membrane 40 (TOMM40)
Gene that codes for a protein responsible for moving proteins into mitochondria.

Traumatic brain injury (TBI)
A head injury causing damage to the brain by external force or mechanism.

Triggering receptor expressed on myeloid cells-2 (TREM2)
Protein that helps regulate removal of cell debris, clearing amyloid proteins and suppressing inflammation in microglia.

Validation therapy
A unique form of therapy that involves listening to elderly seniors with dementia, connecting with them through empathy, and providing dignified care in the last stages of their lives.

Vascular cognitive impairment
A decline in thinking abilities caused by disease that damages the brain's blood vessels.

Vascular dementia
A decline in thinking skills caused by cerebrovascular disease, a condition in which blood vessels in the brain are damaged and brain tissue injured, depriving brain cells of vital oxygen and nutrients.

Verbal memory
The ability to recall words, verbal items, or language-based memories.

Verbal processing
The ability to receive information and ideas through listening and reading, and the ability to send or express information or ideas through speaking and writing.

Visual processing
The brain's ability to use and interpret visual information from the world around us.

Wandering
A behavior that occurs in dementia characterized by a repeated, prolonged, and sometimes compulsive need to walk, with or without aim.

World Health Organization (WHO)
A specialized agency of the United Nations responsible for international public health.

Directory of Resources

ACADEMIC JOURNALS

Alzheimer's & Dementia
Founded and launched in 2005 by the Alzheimer's Association, it is a
monthly publication that shares diverse knowledge about Alzheimer's
science with the global scientific community. A peer-reviewed
journal, *Alzheimer's & Dementia* aims to bridge knowledge gaps
separating traditional fields of dementia research by covering the
entire spectrum, from basic science to clinical trials and social and
behavioral investigations.

Alzheimer's & Dementia: Diagnosis, Assessment, & Disease Monitoring
(*DADM*)
Concentrates on the discovery, development, and validation of assays,
instruments, and technologies with the potential to facilitate accurate detection of dementia in its various forms and stages. Articles
cover a range of topics focused on the early and accurate identification of people at elevated risk of various forms of memory disorders, including individuals who are asymptomatic and those with
memory complaints.

Alzheimer's & Dementia: Translational Research & Clinical Interventions
(*TRCI*)
Seeks to advance and expedite clinical translational research in Alzheimer's disease and age-related cognitive impairment into improved
care and treatment, and promote open-access communication
across preclinical, clinical, and effectiveness research areas. The
journal features findings from diverse domains of research and

disciplines to accelerate the conversion of abstract facts into practical knowledge: specifically, to translate what is learned at the bench into bedside applications.

Journal of Alzheimer's Disease
A peer-reviewed medical journal published by IOS Press covering the etiology, pathogenesis, epidemiology, genetics, treatment, and psychology of Alzheimer's disease.

Psychology and Aging
Publishes original articles that significantly advance knowledge about adult development and aging. The primary focus of the journal is on reports of novel empirical findings that inform theories related to the psychological science of aging and adult development.

BOOKS

The Alzheimer's Society. *How to Help People with Dementia: A Guide for Customer-Facing Staff.* Chicago: Alzheimer's Society, 2014.
  This book explains how small actions can make a big difference when one is serving customers with dementia. A staff member who recognizes symptoms and demonstrates understanding to someone who may be having problems can make that person's day-to-day life much better. This guide is for anyone who works with the general public in a customer-facing role, either face-to-face or providing support via the phone or online channels.
Anderson, Nicole D., Kelly J. Murphy, and Angela K. Troyer. *Living with Mild Cognitive Impairment: A Guide to Maximizing Brain Health and Reducing Risk of Dementia.* New York: Oxford University Press, 2012.
  Specifically for individuals with mild cognitive impairment, for their loved ones, and for the health-care professionals who treat them. Written by three clinicians and researchers who have devoted their careers to MCI patients, this book provides reliable information on the nature of this disorder, how it may affect people, and what can be done about it. The authors explain how MCI is diagnosed and treated and they offer advice on how to improve cognitive health through diet and exercise, through social engagement, and through the use of practical, effective memory strategies.
Coste, Joanne Koenig. *Learning to Speak Alzheimer's: A Groundbreaking Approach for Everyone Dealing with the Disease.* New York: Houghton Mifflin Harcourt Publishing Company, 2004.

Offers a practical approach to the emotional well-being of both patients and caregivers that emphasizes relating to patients in their own reality. The author's accessible and comprehensive method, which she calls "habilitation," works to enhance communication between care partners and patients and has proven successful with thousands of people living with dementia.

Graff-Radford, Jonathon and Angela M. Lunde. *Mayo Clinic on Alzheimer's Disease and Other Dementias: A Guide for People with Dementia and Those Who Care for Them*. New York: Mayo Clinic Press, 2020.

Now in its seventh edition, expert neurologists from the Mayo Clinic organize this new research into a thorough and digestible guidebook that provides caregivers with the most up-to-date information regarding the disease. The book presents a comprehensive look at the typical symptoms associated with dementia and current findings regarding common causes of the disease, and it gives essential tips for managing the day-to-day challenges of caring for someone with dementia.

Gupta, Sanjay. *Keep Sharp: Build a Better Brain at Any Age*. New York: Simon & Schuster, 2021.

Throughout our life, we look for ways to keep our mind sharp and effortlessly productive. Now, globetrotting neurosurgeon Dr. Sanjay Gupta offers insights from top scientists all over the world, whose cutting-edge research can help individuals heighten and protect brain function and maintain cognitive health at any age.

Issacson, Richard S. and Christopher N. Ochner. *The Alzheimer's Prevention and Treatment Diet*. Garden City Park, NY: Square one Publishers, 2016.

Outlines a cutting-edge nutritional program that will be of interest both to Alzheimer's patients and anybody else who wants to maintain optimal memory and mental agility for years to come. The book begins with an overview of Alzheimer's disease, outlining its symptoms, risk factors, diagnosis, and current treatment methods. It also shows how Alzheimer's disease differs from other forms of memory loss and cognitive impairment.

Mace, Nancy L. and Peter V. Rabins. *The 36-Hour Day: The 36-Hour Day: A Family Guide to Caring for People Who Have Alzheimer Disease, Other Dementias, and Memory Loss*. Baltimore, MA: Johns Hopkins University Press, 2017.

An essential resource for families who love and care for people with Alzheimer's disease. Whether a person has Alzheimer's disease or another form of dementia, the person will face a host of problems. This book will help family members and caregivers address these problems and simultaneously cope with their own emotions and needs.

O'Brien, Greg. *On Pluto: Inside the Mind of Alzheimer's.* Brewster, MA: Coldfish Press, 2013.

Greg O'Brien, an award-winning investigative reporter, has been diagnosed with early-onset Alzheimer's and is one of those faceless numbers. Acting on long-term memory and skill coupled with well-developed journalistic grit, O'Brien decided to tackle the disease and his imminent decline by writing frankly about the journey. This is a book about living with Alzheimer's, not dying with it. It is a book about hope, faith, and humor—a prescription far more powerful than the conventional medication available today to fight this disease.

Perlmutter, David with Kristin Loberg. *Grain Brain: The Surprising Truth about Wheat, Carbs, and Sugar—Your Brain's Silent Killers.* New York: Little, Brown Spark, 2018.

Renowned neurologist Perlmutter exposes a finding that has been buried in the medical literature for far too long: carbs are destroying your brain. Even so-called healthy carbs like whole grains can cause dementia, ADHD, epilepsy, anxiety, chronic headaches, depression, decreased libido, and much more. The cornerstone of all degenerative conditions, including brain disorders, is inflammation, which can be triggered by carbs, especially ones that contain gluten or are high in sugar.

Small, Gary and Gigi Vorgan. *The Small Guide to Alzheimer's Disease.* West Palm Beach, FL: Humanix Books, 2020.

Provides readers with an overview of Alzheimer's disease: what it is, who gets it, how to recognize it, and what its major causes (genetics, environment, etc.) are. As best-selling author of *The Memory Bible* and *The Memory Prescription*, as well as director of the UCLA Longevity Center, Dr. Small is on the cutting edge of breakthrough treatments as well as prevention strategies. In addition to case studies and patient interviews, all chapters include sidebars with factoids, lists, and other helpful information.

VIDEOS

"Alzheimer's Is Not Normal Aging, and We Can Cure It" (2015)
https://www.ted.com/talks/samuel_cohen_alzheimer_s_is_not_normal
        _aging_and_we_can_cure_it.

More than 40 million people worldwide suffer from Alzheimer's disease, and that number is expected to increase drastically in the coming years. But no real progress has been made in the fight against the disease since its classification more than 100 years ago. Scientist Samuel Cohen shares a new breakthrough in Alzheimer's research from his lab as well as a message of hope. "Alzheimer's is a disease," Cohen says, "and we can cure it."

"The Brain Changing Benefits to Exercising" (2017)
https://www.ted.com/talks/wendy_suzuki_the_brain_changing_benefits _of_exercise.
What's the most transformative thing that you can do for your brain today? Exercise! according to neuroscientist Wendy Suzuki. Get inspired to go to the gym as Suzuki discusses the science of how working out boosts your mood and memory—and protects your brain against neurodegenerative diseases such as Alzheimer's.

"The Coming Neurological Epidemic" (2008)
https://www.ted.com/talks/gregory_petsko_the_coming_neurological _epidemic.
Biochemist Gregory Petsko makes a convincing argument that, in the next 50 years, we'll see an epidemic of neurological diseases, such as Alzheimer's, as the world population ages. His solution: more research into the brain and its functions.

"Could Your Brain Repair Itself?" (2015)
https://www.ted.com/talks/ralitsa_petrova_could_your_brain_repair_itself.
Imagine the brain could reboot, updating its damaged cells with new, improved units. That may sound like science fiction, but it's a potential reality scientists are investigating right now. Ralitsa Petrova details the science behind neurogenesis and explains how we might harness it to reverse diseases such as Alzheimer's and Parkinson's.

The Forgetting: A Portrait of Alzheimer's (2004)
https://www.pbs.org/video/january-16-2004-24373/.
This 90-minute Emmy Award-winning documentary that first aired on PBS follows the stories of several patients and their families. It also weaves in the biology of the disease and the attempts to find a cure.

"How I'm Preparing to Get Alzheimer's Disease" (2012)
https://www.ted.com/talks/alanna_shaikh_how_i_m_preparing_to_get _alzheimer_s.
When faced with a parent suffering from Alzheimer's, most of us respond with denial ("It won't happen to me") or extreme efforts at prevention. But global health expert and TED Fellow Alanna Shaikh sees

it differently. She's taking three concrete steps to prepare for the moment—should it arrive—when she herself gets Alzheimer's disease.

Sum Total of Our Memory: Facing Alzheimer's Together (2014)
http://thesumtotalmovie.com
Couples affected by a partner's recent diagnosis of Early Alzheimer's come to terms with their changing roles. Prominent Alzheimer's medical experts offer their perspectives on diagnosis, the nature of the disease, helpful attitudes in caring for loved ones, stigma, clinical trials, support for caregivers, and overall health-care concerns.

"What You Can Do To Prevent Alzheimer's" (2017)
https://www.ted.com/talks/lisa_genova_what_you_can_do_to_prevent_alzheimer_s?language=en.
Alzheimer's doesn't have to be your brain's destiny, says neuroscientist and author of *Still Alice*, Lisa Genova. She shares the latest science investigating the disease—and some promising research on what each of us can do to build an Alzheimer's-resistant brain.

"What's the Connection between Sleep and Alzheimer's Disease?" (2020)
https://www.ted.com/talks/matt_walker_what_s_the_connection_between_sleep_and_alzheimer_s_disease.
Does not getting enough sleep lead to Alzheimer's disease? Sleep scientist Matt Walker explains the relationship between the two—and how researchers are exploring how to use sleep to decrease our chances of developing this condition.

WEBSITES

ALZFORUM: Networking for a Cure
https://www.alzforum.org.
Founded in 1996, Alzforum is a news website and information resource dedicated to helping researchers accelerate discovery and advance development of diagnostics and treatments for Alzheimer's disease and related disorders.

Alzheimer's Association
http://www.alz.org.
This comprehensive site provides information on warning signs, stages of the disease, treatments, care options, and financial planning. ALZConnected offers chat rooms for those diagnosed with the

disease and for caregivers. You also can find local support groups for caregivers and individuals with younger-onset and early-stage Alzheimer's. Check the community resource finder for information on local services. With its caregiver center, you can enter information about an individual's medical condition and needs, and a personalized printout will offer recommendations about care options.

Alzheimer's Association's Alzheimer's and Dementia Caregiver Center
https://www.alz.org/help-support/caregiving.
The Alzheimer's and Dementia Caregiver Center is the Alzheimer's Association's caregiver portal, providing a window into a variety of tools and resources. There you'll find help on behaviors, communication, legal and financial matters, and care options, as well as tips on driving and safety issues, activities for your loved one, and respite care. This site is a point of reference you will likely return to time and time again.

Alzheimer's Association's Alzheimer's Navigator
https://www.alzheimersnavigator.org.
When facing Alzheimer's disease, there are a lot of things to consider. Alzheimer's Navigator helps guide caregivers to answers by creating a personalized action plan and providing links to information, support, and local resources.

Alzheimer's Association's Care Training Resources
https://www.alz.org/help-support/resources/care-training-resources.
Being a caregiver doesn't come with an instruction manual, but there are resources available to help. Use the free trainings and workshops on this site to gain caregiving skills and practical advice.

Alzheimer's Association's 24/7 Helpline (800) 272-3900
https://www.alz.org/help-support/resources/helpline.
When you're in the midst of a crisis, dementia caregivers can call the Alzheimer's Association's Helpline 24 hours a day, 7 days per week to talk to master's-level clinicians and specialists. This helpline offers crisis guidance, decision support, education, information on local programs and services, information on financial and legal resources, treatment options, and care decisions. There's also a live internet chat option available from 7:00 a.m. to 7:00 p.m., Monday through Friday. The Alzheimer's Association offers plenty of downloadable resources, too, covering many questions and concerns that dementia caregivers face.

By Us For Us Guides

https://the-ria.ca/resources/by-us-for-us-guides.

PDF guides created through the Kenneth G. Murray Alzheimer Research and Education Program (MAREP) at the University of Waterloo by persons with dementia for persons with dementia. The guides are practical tools to help enhance well-being and manage daily challenges.

Centers for Disease Control and Prevention: Healthy Brain Initiative

https://www.cdc.gov/aging/healthybrain.

The Healthy Brain Initiative improves understanding of brain health as a central part of public health practice. The initiative creates and supports partnerships, collects and reports data, increases awareness of brain health, supports populations with a high burden of Alzheimer's disease and related dementias, and promotes the use of its Road Map series. The Road Map series provides actionable steps to promote brain health, address cognitive impairment, and address the needs of caregivers.

Community Resource Finder

https://www.communityresourcefinder.org.

Community Resource Finder is an Alzheimer's Association tool that will help you locate resources, services, and programs right in your own community. It's as simple as entering your zip code and choosing from a list of over 20 categories, including eldercare attorneys, assisted living communities, area agencies on aging, home health care, and more. The site also provides various links back to many other Alzheimer's Association resources.

Dementia Friendly America

https://www.dfamerica.org.

Dementia Friendly America is "a national network of communities, organizations, and individuals seeking to ensure that communities across the United States are equipped to support people living with dementia and their caregivers." DFA offers a robust list of resources for people living with dementia, their loved ones, and dementia caregivers, as well as toolkits for those who want to advocate in their own communities.

Dementia Support Group Searchable Database

https://www.alz.org/events/event_search.

Support groups are some of the best resources available to dementia caregivers. Connecting with other caregivers who are going through similar journeys and experiences helps caregivers feel as though they're not alone. And other caregivers are often excellent sources of advice for dealing with specific caregiving situations. The Alzheimer's Association offers a searchable database of support groups, making it easy for caregivers who want to join an in-person group to find a support group in their local area.

Eldercare Workforce Alliance: Caregiver Resources
https://eldercareworkforce.org/resources/caregiver-resources.
The Eldercare Workforce Alliance is a group of 35 national organizations joined together to address the immediate and future workforce crisis in caring for an aging America. Their mission is to build a caring and competent eldercare workforce, joining in partnership with older adults, their families, and other unpaid caregivers, to provide high-quality, culturally sensitive, person-directed, family-focused care and to improve the quality of life for older adults and their families.

Family Caregiver Alliance: Dementia Caregiver Resources
https://www.caregiver.org/caregiver-resources/health-conditions/dementia.
The Family Caregiver Alliance provides an abundance of resources for caregivers to people with a variety of health conditions and disabilities. The Dementia Caregiver Resources section is a trove of helpful guides, tip sheets, and caregiver stories to help caregivers navigate the journey of caring for a loved one with dementia. The Family Caregiver Alliance also offers online support groups for caregivers to connect with others who are facing similar struggles and those who can offer advice for overcoming common caregiving challenges.

Fisher Center for Alzheimer's Research Foundation
www.alzinfo.org.
This wide-ranging site provides information on the latest research, treatments, and exercises to keep mentally fit. Read blogs by caregivers, researchers, and persons with the disease. The "Ask the Expert" feature enables you to submit questions to researchers. With its resource locator, you can find nearby medical suppliers, physical therapists, geriatric physicians, elder law attorneys, and other resources.

The Hartford: Dementia and Driving
https://www.thehartford.com/resources/mature-market-excellence/dementia-driving.

The insurer provides information on the impact of dementia on driving safety. It offers tips on evaluating one's driving skills, information on safety technologies and pointers to family members on how to persuade those with impairments to stop driving.

Healthy Brains
https://healthybrains.org.
The Cleveland Clinic's Healthy Brains initiative offers individualized brain health assessment tools, lifestyle tips, news on the latest developments in research and medicine, and more. This interactive resource is useful for both caregivers and those who are living with Alzheimer's disease or another form of dementia, offering both tips for reducing the risk of developing dementia as well as helpful resources for caregivers, such as information on the healing power of pets, the latest clinical trials, and more.

Mayo Clinic: Relaxation Techniques
https://www.mayoclinic.org/healthy-lifestyle/stress-management/in -depth/relaxation-technique/art-20045368.
Relaxation techniques are a great way to help with stress management. Relaxation isn't only about peace of mind or enjoying a hobby. Relaxation is a process that decreases the effects of stress on your mind and body.

Memory Cafés
https://www.memorycafedirectory.com.
Located in hospitals, libraries, senior centers, and other locations, memory cafés offer support for those with dementia and their caregivers to help them combat social isolation and connect with others who are coping with similar circumstances. The Memory Café directory lists hundreds of memory cafés located throughout the United States.

National Alliance for Caregiving: Brain Health Conversation Guide
https://www.caregiving.org/wp-content/uploads/2020/05/TalkBrain Health_Nov-1-2016.pdf.
The National Alliance for Caregiving offers support and resources for all caregivers, but dementia caregivers will find the Brain Health Conversation Guide, developed in collaboration with the Alzheimer's Foundation of America, particularly helpful for navigating those difficult discussions about memory changes and cognitive health. Talking about brain health does not have to be scary. This guide can help you start a conversation about those

changes. Use it to talk with family, close friends, and health-care professionals.

National Institute on Aging: Alzheimer's Disease Diagnostic Guidelines
https://www.nia.nih.gov/health/alzheimers-disease-diagnostic-guidelines.
This website provides detailed information and updates for health professionals.

National Institute on Aging: Alzheimer's Disease Education and Referral Center
https://www.nia.nih.gov/health/alzheimers.
Providing information on the latest studies on causes and possible cures, the database can be searched for publications, research centers, and clinical trials. This extensive, consumer-friendly site offers science-based advice on nutrition, exercise, treatment, and prevention, and the ability to download or order a free copy of NIA's excellent 104-page *Caring for a Person with Alzheimer's Disease.*

National Institute on Aging: Dementia Research and Clinical Trials
https://www.nia.nih.gov/health/alzheimers/dementia-research-and -clinical-trials.
Scientists are making great strides in identifying potential new ways to help diagnose, treat, and even prevent Alzheimer's and related dementias. These advances are possible because thousands of people have participated in clinical trials and other studies.

National Institute on Aging: Next Steps after a Diagnosis of Alzheimer's Disease
https://www.nia.nih.gov/health/next-steps-after-alzheimers-diagnosis.
This handout, created for prospective patients, provides a wealth of information and resources about health care, safety, and more. Available in English and Spanish.

A Place for Mom: The Big List of Alzheimer's Resources
https://www.aplaceformom.com/blog/list-of-alzheimers-resources-3 -06-2013.
The Big List of Alzheimer's Resources from A Place for Mom will steer you to resources on everything from clinical trials and genetic testing to video, book, and blog recommendations. You'll also find links to wonderful sites offering caregiver support and providing news on the latest research developments, prevention tips, and even music therapy. The Big List makes a great jumping-off point if you're new to the world of Alzheimer's and dementia.

Reddit.com: Alzheimer's Disease

https://www.reddit.com/r/Alzheimers.

R/alzheimers is a popular internet forum for people effected by Alzheimer's disease and dementia to support one another and share news about these conditions.

SAGE Test: 15 Minute At-Home Test for Alzheimer's

https://dailycaring.com/sage-test-for-alzheimers-at-home.

If you suspect that your older adult is having problems with memory, thinking, or judgement, you may want them to take the SAGE test for dementia. This at-home pen-and-paper test is free, takes just 15 minutes, and accurately identifies early symptoms of Alzheimer's or dementia. Studies confirming the validity of the test have found that the test can identify 80% of people with mild cognition and memory issues. Among people who do not have cognition issues, 95% will have normal scores.

This Caring Home

http://www.thiscaringhome.org.

Click on a room in a virtual house, and you will read about safety recommendations. The site also lists room-by-room solutions for dozens of common problems, from forgetting to close a refrigerator door to toileting issues. The site has reviewed numerous products, such as faucet devices that prevent scalding, memory aids, and automatic stovetop fire extinguishers.

University of Washington Alzheimer's Disease Research Center: Mini-Course: Alzheimer's Disease and Related Dementias

https://depts.washington.edu/mbwc/adrc/page/ADRD-mini-course.

The course includes four video presentations and companion slides, and covers healthy and unhealthy brain aging, clinical essentials of Alzheimer's disease and related dementias, vascular brain injury, and a research framework for Alzheimer's disease and related dementias.

U.S. Department of Veterans Affairs: Dementia Care

https://www.va.gov/GERIATRICS/pages/Alzheimers_and_Dementia_Care.asp.

For dementia caregivers providing care for a veteran, the U.S. Department of Veterans Affairs offers helpful information on Alzheimer's disease and other dementias, as well as information on the services and resources available to veterans living with dementia. Services provided include support for both veterans and their caregivers.

WebMD: Alzheimer's Disease and Financial Planning
https://www.webmd.com/alzheimers/guide/financial-planning#1.
In addition to the site's wealth of medical advice about Alzheimer's and
      dementia, WebMD offers a guide on financial considerations with
      regard to Alzheimer's disease. It provides basic information about
      options for paying for long-term care, including health and disabil-
      ity insurance, Medicare, and Medicaid.

World Health Organization
http://www.who.int/en.
Working through offices in more than 150 countries, WHO staff work side
      by side with governments and other partners to ensure the highest
      attainable level of health for all people.

Bibliography

Alber, Jessica, Danielle Goldfarb, Louisa I. Thompson, Edmund Arthur, Kimberly Hernandez, Derrick Cheng, Delia Cabrera DeBuc, et al. "Developing Retinal Biomarkers for the Earliest Stages of Alzheimer's Disease: What We Know, What We Don't, and How to Move Forward." *Alzheimer's & Dementia: The Journal of the Alzheimer's Association* 16, no. 1 (2020): 229–243. https://doi.org/10.1002/alz.12006.

Alzheimer's Association. "Guide to Memory Loss Concerns." https://alz.org/alzheimers-dementia/memory-loss-concerns.

Alzheimer's Association. "Issues Brief: LGBT and Dementia." August 2018. https://www.sageusa.org/resource-posts/issues-brief-lgbt-and-dementia.

Alzheimer's Association. "Research and Progress: Milestones." https://www.alz.org/alzheimers-dementia/research_progress/milestones.

"Alzheimer's Disease Fact Sheet." National Institute on Aging, May 22, 2019. https://www.nia.nih.gov/health/alzheimers-disease-fact-sheet.

"Alzheimer's May Soon Be Predicted during Eye Exams." Neuroscience News, August 23, 2018. https://neurosciencenews.com/eye-exam-alzheimers-9732.

"Alzheimer's Memory Loss Reversed by New Head Device Using Electromagnetic Waves." *Neuroscience News*, September 17, 2019. https://neurosciencenews.com/alzheimers-memory-electromagnetic-waves-14920.

"Alzheimer 'Tau' Protein Far Surpasses Amyloid in Predicting Toll on Brain Tissue." *UC San Francisco*, January 1, 2020. https://www.ucsf.edu/news/2019/12/416296/alzheimer-tau-protein-far-surpasses-amyloid-predicting-toll-brain-tissue.

American Association of Nurse Practitioners. "NP Fact Sheet." August 2020. https://www.aanp.org/all-about-nps/np-fact-sheet.

American Psychiatric Association. "About *DSM-5.*" Psychiatry.org, 2019. https://www.psychiatry.org/psychiatrists/practice/dsm/about-dsm.

Andrews, Megan, Babak Tousi, and Marwan N. Sabbagh. "5HT6 Antagonists in the Treatment of Alzheimer's Dementia: Current Progress." *Neurology and Therapy* 7, no. 1 (2018): 51–58. https://doi.org/10.1007 /s40120-018-0095-y.

Arthur, Paul B., Laura N. Gitlin, John A. Kairalla, and William C. Mann. "Relationship between the Number of Behavioral Symptoms in Dementia and Caregiver Distress: What Is the Tipping Point?" *International Psychogeriatrics* 30, no. 8 (2018): 1099–1107. https://doi .org/10.1017/S104161021700237X.

Atri, Alireza. "Current and Future Treatments in Alzheimer's Disease." *Seminars in Neurology* 39, no. 2 (2019): 227–240. https://doi.org /10.1055/s-0039-1678581.

Belluck, Pam. "Will We Ever Cure Alzheimer's?" *New York Times*, November 20, 2018. https://www.nytimes.com/2018/11/19/health /dementia-alzheimers-cure-drugs.html.

Bevan-Jones, W. Richard, Thomas E. Cope, P. Simon Jones, Sanne S. Kaalund, Luca Passamonti, Kieren Allinson, Oliver Green, et al. "Neuroinflammation and Protein Aggregation Co-Localize across the Frontotemporal Dementia Spectrum." *Brain* 143, no. 1 (2020): 1010–1026. https://doi.org/10.1093/brain/awaa033.

Bird, Thomas D. "Alzheimer Disease Overview." In GeneReviews® [Internet], edited by M. P. Adam, H. H. Ardinger, R. A. Pagon, et al. Seattle: University of Washington, updated December 20, 2018. https:// www.ncbi.nlm.nih.gov/books/NBK1161.

Birks, Jacqueline S. "Cholinesterase Inhibitors for Alzheimer's Disease." *Cochrane Database of Systematic Reviews* 25, no. 1 (2006): 25. https://doi.org/10.1002/14651858.CD005593.

"Blood Test Enables Early Diagnosis of Alzheimer's Disease." Lund University, September 15, 2020. https://www.lunduniversity.lu.se/article /new-blood-test-detecting-alzheimers-disease.

"Body Clock Disruptions Occur Years before Memory Loss in Alzheimer's." *ScienceDaily*, January 29, 2018. http://www.sciencedaily.com /releases/2018/01/180129150033.htm.

Bondi, Mark W., Emily C. Edmonds, and David P. Salmon. "Alzheimer's Disease: Past, Present, and Future." *Journal of the International Neuropsychological Society* 23, no. 9–10 (2017): 818–831. https:// doi.org/10.1017/s135561771700100x.

"Brain and Brawn: Hitting the Gym Slows Neurodegeneration in Older People at Risk of Alzheimer's." *Neuroscience from Technology Networks*, February 17, 2020. https://www.technologynetworks

.com/neuroscience/news/brain-and-brawn-hitting-the-gym-slows
-neurodegeneration-in-older-people-at-risk-of-alzheimers-330905.

"The Brain May Clean out Alzheimer's Plaques during Sleep." *Science News*, July 15, 2018. http://www.sciencenews.org/article/sleep-brain-alzheimers-plaques-protein.

"Brain 'Pacemaker' Gives Hope to Alzheimer's Patients." Barrow Neurological Foundation, September 13, 2019. https://www.supportbarrow.org/news/brain-pacemaker-gives-hope-to-alzheimers-patients.

"Brain Scans and Dementia." Stanford Health Care. https://stanfordhealthcare.org/medical-conditions/brain-and-nerves/dementia/diagnosis/brain-scans.html.

Bubu, Omonigho M., Michael Brannick, James Mortimer, Ogie Umasabor-Bubu, Yuri V. Sebastião, Yi Wen, Skai Schwartz, et al. "Sleep, Cognitive Impairment, and Alzheimer's Disease: A Systematic Review and Meta-Analysis." *Sleep* 40, no. 1 (2016): 1–18. https://doi.org/10.1093/sleep/zsw032.

Buchman, A. S., P. A. Boyle, L. Yu, R. C. Shah, R. S. Wilson, and D. A. Bennett. "Total Daily Physical Activity and the Risk of AD and Cognitive Decline in Older Adults." *Neurology* 78, no. 17 (2012): 1323–1329. https://doi.org/10.1212/WNL.0b013e3182535d35.

Burke, Anna, Geri R. Hall, Roy Yaari, Adam Fleisher, Jan Dougherty, Jeffrey Young, Helle Brand, and Pierre Tariot. *Pocket Reference to Alzheimer's Disease Management*. London: Springer Healthcare, 2015.

Caruso, Alessandra, Ferdinando Nicoletti, Alessandra Gaetano, and Sergio Scaccianoce. "Risk Factors for Alzheimer's Disease: Focus on Stress." *Frontiers in Pharmacology* 10 (2019). https://doi.org/10.3389/fphar.2019.00976.

Castro, Diego M., Carol Dillon, Gerardo Machnicki, and Ricardo F. Allegri. "The Economic Cost of Alzheimer's Disease: Family or Public Health Burden?" *Dementia & Neuropsychologia* 4, no. 4 (2010): 262–267. https://doi.org/10.1590/S1980-57642010DN40400003.

Chan, John S. Y., Kanfeng Deng, Jiamin Wu, and Jin H Yan. "Effects of Meditation and Mind–Body Exercises on Older Adults' Cognitive Performance: A Meta-Analysis." *The Gerontologist* 16, no. 59 (2019): e782–e790. https://doi.org/10.1093/geront/gnz022.

Cheng, Sheung-Tak. "Cognitive Reserve and the Prevention of Dementia: the Role of Physical and Cognitive Activities." *Current Psychiatry Reports* 18, no. 9 (2016): 85. https://doi.org/10.1007/s11920-016-0721-2.

Chiba-Falek, Ornit, William K. Gottschalk, and Micahel W. Lutz. "The Effects of the TOMM40 poly-T Alleles on Alzheimer's Disease

Phenotypes." *Alzheimer's & Dementia: The Journal of the Alzheimer's Association* 14, no. 5 (2018): 692–698. https://doi.org/10.1016/j.jalz.2018.01.015.

Cipriani, Gabriele, Cristina Dolciotti, Lucia Picchi, and Ubaldo Bonuccelli. "Alzheimer and His Disease: A Brief History." *Neurological Sciences* 32, no. 2 (2011): 275–279. https://doi.org/10.1007/s10072-010-0454-7.

Cohut, Maria. "Future of Alzheimer's Therapy: What Is the Best Approach?" *Medical News Today*, December 10, 2018. https://www.medicalnewstoday.com/articles/323944.

"Could Reducing Brain Inflammation Prevent Memory Loss in Alzheimer's?" *Medical News Today*, March 26, 2020. https://www.medicalnewstoday.com/articles/could-reducing-brain-inflammation-prevent-memory-loss-in-alzheimers.

Creswell, David J. "Mindfulness Interventions." *Annual Review of Psychology* 68, no. 1 (2017): 491–516. https://doi.org/10.1146/annurev-psych-042716-051139.

Cummings, Jeffrey L., Gary Tong, and Clive Ballard. "Treatment Combinations for Alzheimer's Disease: Current and Future Pharmacotherapy Options." *Journal of Alzheimer's Disease* 67, no. 3 (2019): 779–794. https://doi.org/10.3233/jad-180766.

Dallemagne, Patrick and Christophe Rochais. "Facing the Complexity of Alzheimer's Disease." *Future Medicinal Chemistry* 12, no. 3 (2020): 175–177. https://doi.org/10.4155/fmc-2019-0310.

Dassel, Kara B. and Dawn C. Carr. "Does Dementia Caregiving Accelerate Frailty? Findings from the Health and Retirement Study." *Gerontologist* 56, no. 3 (2016): 444–450. https://doi.org/10.1093/geront/gnu078.

"Definitions for GERAS." Definitions.com. https://www.definitions.net/definition/GERAS.

"Dementia Caregiving in the U.S." National Alliance for Caregiving, in partnership with the Alzheimer's Association, October 2017. https://www.caregiving.org/wp-content/uploads/2020/05/Dementia-Caregiving-Report-2017_Research-Recommendations_FINAL.pdf.

Devore, Elizabeth E., Jae Hee Kang, Monique M. B. Breteler, and Francine Grodstein. "Dietary Intakes of Berries and Flavonoids in Relation to Cognitive Decline." *Annals of Neurology* 72, no. 1 (2012): 135–143. https://doi.org/10.1002/ana.23594.

"Diet and Alzheimer's: Symptoms Reduced in Lab Models." USC News, March 6, 2019. https://news.usc.edu/154890/alzheimers-like-symptoms-in-mice-reversed-with-special-diet.

Donix, Marcus, Gary W. Small, and Susan Y. Bookheimer. "Family History and APOE-4 Genetic Risk in Alzheimer's Disease." *Neuropsychology*

Review 22 (2012): 298–309. https://doi.org/10.1007/s11065-012 -9193-2.

"Eating More Ketones May Fight against Alzheimer's Disease." Neuroscience News, December 9, 2019. https://neurosciencenews.com /alzheimers-ketones-15301.

Ertel, Karen, Maria Glymour, and Lisa Berkman. "Effects of Social Integration on Preserving Memory Function in a Nationally Representative US Elderly Population." *American Journal of Public Health* 98, no. 7 (2008): 1215–1220.

"Exercise Could Slow Withering Effects of Alzheimer's." Neuroscience News, September 17, 2019. https://neurosciencenews.com/alzheimers -exercise-14924.

Feil, Naomi. *The Validation Breakthrough: Simple Techniques for Communication with People with Alzheimer's Type Dementia.* Baltimore, MD: Health Professions Press, 1993.

Ferreira-Vieira, Talita H., Isabella M. Guimaraes, Flavia R. Silva, and Fabiola M. Ribeiro. "Alzheimer's Disease: Targeting the Cholinergic System." *Current Neuropharmacology* 14, no. 1 (2016): 101–115. https://doi.org/10.2174/1570159x13666150716165726.

Fischman, Josh. "The Future of Medicine: A New Era for Alzheimer's." *Scientific American*, May 2020.

Foley, Katherine Ellen. "The Future of Alzheimer's Treatment Can't Bank on Just One Drug." *Quartz*, October 24, 2019. https://qz.com /1734078/the-future-of-alzheimers-treatment-cant-bank-on-just -one-drug.

Forbes, Dorothy, Ivan Culum, Andrea R. Lischka, Debra G. Morgan, Shelley Peacock, Jennifer Forbes, and Sean Forbes. "Light Therapy for Managing Cognitive, Sleep, Functional, Behavioural, or Psychiatric Disturbances in Dementia." *Cochrane Database of Systematic Reviews* 4, no. 1 (2009): CD003946. https://doi.org/10.1002/14651858 .CD003946.pub3.

Fredman, Lisa, Rosanna M. Bertrand, Lynn M. Martire, Marc Hochberg, and Emily L. Harris. "Leisure-Time Exercise and Overall Physical Activity in Older Women Caregivers and Non-Caregivers from the Caregiver-SOF Study." *Preventive Medicine* 43, no. 3 (2006): 226–229. https://doi.org/10.1016/j.ypmed.2006.04.009.

Fried, Itzhak. "Brain Stimulation in Alzheimer's Disease." *Journal of Alzheimer's Disease* 54, no. 2 (2016): 789–791. https://pubmed.ncbi .nlm.nih.gov/27567879.

Friedman, Esther M., Regina A. Shih, Kenneth M. Langa, and Michael D. Hurd. "US Prevalence and Predictors of Informal Caregiving for Dementia." *Health Affairs* 34, no. 10 (2015): 1637–1641. https://doi .org/10.1377/hlthaff.2015.0510.

Gao, Chenlu, Nikita Y. Chapagain, and Michael K. Scullin. "Sleep Duration and Sleep Quality in Caregivers of Patients with Dementia: A Systematic Review and Meta-Analysis." *JAMA Network Open* 2, no. 8 (2019): e199891. https://doi.org/10.1001/jamanetworkopen.2019.9891.

Garity, Joan. "Caring for a Family Member with Alzheimer's Disease: Coping with Caregiver Burden Post–Nursing Home Placement." *Journal of Gerontological Nursing* 32, no. 6 (2006): 39–48. https://doi.org/10.3928/00989134-20060601-07.

Gitlin, Laura N. and Nancy Hodgson. "Caregivers as Therapeutic Agents in Dementia Care: The Evidence-Base for Interventions Supporting Their Role." In *Family Caregiving in the New Normal*, edited by J. E. Gaugler and R. L. Kane, 305–356. Philadelphia: Elsevier, 2015.

Gitlin, Laura N., Katherine Marx, Ian H. Stanley, and Nancy Hodgson. "Translating Evidence-Based Dementia Caregiving Interventions into Practice: State-of-the-Science and Next Steps." *The Gerontologist* 55, no. 2 (2015): 210–226. https://doi.org/10.1093/geront/gnu123.

Gong, C. X. and K. Iqbal. "Hyperphosphorylation of Microtubule-Associated Protein Tau: A Promising Therapeutic Target for Alzheimer Disease." *Current Medicinal Chemistry* 5, no. 23 (2008): 2321–2328. https://doi.org/10.2174/092986708785909111.

Graff-Radford, Jonathon and Angela M. Lunde. *Mayo Clinic on Alzheimer's Disease and Other Dementias: A Guide for People with Dementia and Those Who Care for Them.* New York: RosettaBooks, 2020.

Grammatikopoulou, Maria G., Dimitrios G. Goulis, Konstantinos Gkiouras, Xenophon Theodoridis, Kalliopi K. Gkouskou, Athanasios Evangeliou, Efthimis Dardiotis, et al. "To Keto or Not to Keto? A Systematic Review of Randomized Controlled Trials Assessing the Effects of Ketogenic Therapy on Alzheimer Disease." *Advances in Nutrition* 11, no. 6 (November 2020): 1583–1602. https://doi.org/10.1093/advances/nmaa073.

Gratuze, Maud, Cheryl E. G. Leyns, and David M. Holtzman. "New Insights into the Role of TREM2 in Alzheimer's Disease." *Molecular Neurodegeneration* 13, no. 66 (2018). https://doi.org/10.1186/s13024-018-0298-9.

Greenwood, Nan and Raymond Smith. "Motivations for Being Informal Carers of People Living with Dementia: A Systematic Review of Qualitative Literature." *BMC Geriatrics* 19, no. 1 (2019): Article 169. https://doi.org/10.1186/s12877-019-1185-0.

Harding, Anne. "Diabetes Doubles Alzheimer's Risk." CNN Digital, September 19, 2011. http://www.cnn.com/2011/09/19/health/diabetes-doubles-alzheimers/index.html.

Harrison, Ian F., Asif Machhada, Niall Colgan, Ozama Ismail, James M. O'Callaghan, Holly Holmes, Jack A. Wells, et al. "P2-150: Glymphatic Clearance Impaired in a Mouse Model of Tauopathy: Captured Using Contrast-Enhanced MRI." *Alzheimer's & Dementia* 11, no. 7 (July 2015): P544. https://doi.org/10.1016/j.jalz.2015.06 .688.

"Healthy Lifestyle May Offset Genetic Risk of Dementia." Neuroscience News, July 14, 2019. https://neurosciencenews.com/lifestyle -genetics-alzheimers-14480.

Hebert, Liesi E., Laurel A. Beckett, Paul A. Scherr, and Denis A. Evans. "Annual Incidence of Alzheimer Disease in the United States Projected to the Years 2000 through 2050." *Alzheimer Disease and Associated Disorders* 15, no. 4 (2001): 169–173. https://doi .org/10.1097/00002093-200110000-00002.

Hebert, L. E., J. Weuve, P. A. Scherr, and D. A. Evans. "Alzheimer Disease in the United States (2010–2050) Estimated Using the 2010 Census." *Neurology* 8, no. 19 (2013): 1778–1783. https://doi.org/10.1212 /wnl.0b013e31828726f5.

Heerema, Esther. "Differences between Delirium and Dementia." Very Well Health. Medically reviewed by Nicholas R. Metrus, MD, on January 25, 2020. https://www.verywellhealth.com/whats-the -difference-between-delirium-and-dementia-98838.

Hemonnot, Anne-Laure, Jennifer Hua, Lauriane Ulmann, and Hélène Hirbec. "Microglia in Alzheimer Disease: Well-Known Targets and New Opportunities." *Frontiers in Aging Neuroscience* 11 (2019): 233. https://doi.org/10.3389/fnagi.2019.00233.

Henderson, Samuel T., Janet L. Vogel, Linda J. Barr, Fiona Garvin, Julie J. Jones, and Lauren C. Costantini. "Study of the Ketogenic Agent AC-1202 in Mild to Moderate Alzheimer's Disease: A Randomized, Double-Blind, Placebo-Controlled, Multicenter Trial." *Nutrition & Metabolism* 6, no. 31 (2009): 1–25. https://doi.org/10.1186/1743 -7075-6-31.

Heutz, Rachel. "Can Mindfulness Beat Alzheimer's Disease?" *Maastricht Journal of Liberal Arts* 9, no. 27 (2017): 33. https://doi.org/10.26481 /mjla.2017.v9.453.

Hippius, Hanns and Gabriele Neundörfer. "The Discovery of Alzheimer's Disease." *Dialogues in Clinical Neuroscience* 5, no. 1 (2003): 101–108. https://doi.org/10.31887/DCNS.2003.5.1/hhippius.

Howe, Edmund G. "Ethical Issues in Diagnosing and Treating Alzheimer's Disease." *Psychiatry* 3, no. 5 (2006): 43–53.

Hudomiet, Péter, Michael D Hurd, and Susann Rohwedder. "Dementia Prevalence in the United States in 2000 and 2012: Estimates Based on a Nationally Representative Study." *Journals of Gerontology*

Series B 73, suppl. 1 (May 2018): S10–19. https://doi.org/10.1093 /geronb/gbx169.

Husna Ibrahim, Nurul, Mohamad Fairuz Yahaya, Wael Mohamed, Seong Lin Teoh, Chua Kien Hui, and Jaya Kumar. "Pharmacotherapy of Alzheimer's Disease: Seeking Clarity in a Time of Uncertainty." *Frontiers in Pharmacology* 11, no. 24 (2020). https://doi.org/10.3389 /fphar.2020.00261.

Iacono, Diego, Peter Zandi, Myron Gross, William R. Markesbery, Olga Pletnikova, Gay Rudow, and Juan C. Troncoso. "APOε2 and Education in Cognitively Normal Older Subjects with High Levels of AD Pathology at Autopsy: Findings from the Nun Study." *Oncotarget* 6, no. 16 (2015): 14082–14091. https://doi.org/10.18632/oncotarget .4118.

Insel, Philip S., Michael Weiner, R. Scott Mackin, Elizabeth Mormino, Yen Y. Lim, Erik Stomrud, Sebastian Palmqvist, et al. "Determining Clinically Meaningful Decline in Preclinical Alzheimer Disease." *Neurology* 93, no. 4 (2019): e322–e333. https://doi.org/10.1212 /WNL.0000000000007831.

Institute of Medicine. *Retooling for an Aging America: Building the Health Care Workforce.* Washington, DC: National Academies Press, 2008. https://doi.org/10.17226/12089.

Janelidze, Shorena, Niklas Mattsson, Sebastian Palmqvist, Ruben Smith, Thomas G. Beach, Geidy E. Serrano, Xiyun Chai, et al. "Plasma P-Tau181 in Alzheimer's Disease: Relationship to Other Biomarkers, Differential Diagnosis, Neuropathology and Longitudinal Progression to Alzheimer's Dementia." *Nature Medicine* 26, no. 3 (2020): 379–386. https://doi.org/10.1038/s41591-020-0755-1.

Jessen, Nadia Aalling, Anne Sofie Finmann Munk, Iben Lundgaard, and Maiken Nedergaard. "The Glymphatic System: A Beginner's Guide." *Neurochemical Research* 40, no. 12 (2015): 2583–2599. https://doi .org/10.1007/s11064-015-1581-6.

Johnson, Gail V. W. and William H. Stoothoff. "Tau Phosphorylation in Neuronal Cell Function and Dysfunction." *Journal of Cell Science* 117 (2004): 5721–5729. https://doi.org/10.1242/jcs.01558.

Jutkowitz, Eric, Robert L. Kane, Joseph E. Gaugler, Richard F. MacLehose, Bryan Dowd, and Karen M. Kuntz. "Societal and Family Lifetime Cost of Dementia: Implications for Policy." *Journal of the American Geriatrics Society* 65, no. 10 (2017): 2169–2175. https://doi.org /10.1111/jgs.15043.

Kasper, Judith D., Vicki A. Freedman, and Brenda C. Spillman. "Disability and Care Needs of Older Americans by Dementia Status: An Analysis of the 2011 National Health and Aging Trends Study." U.S. Department of Health and Human Services, 2014. http://aspe.hhs

.gov/report/disability-and-care-needs-older-americans-dementia
-status-analysis-2011-national-health-and-aging-trends-study.

Khatutsky, Galina, Joshua Wiener, Wayne Anderson, Valentina Akhmerova, Andrew Jessup, and Marie R. Squillace. "Understanding Direct Care Workers: A Snapshot of Two of America's Most Important Jobs: Certified Nursing Assistants and Home Health Aides." U.S. Department of Health and Human Services, March, 2011. https://aspe.hhs.gov/basic-report/understanding-direct-care -workers-snapshot-two-americas-most-important-jobs-certified -nursing-assistants-and-home-health-aides.

Lange, Klaus W., Katharina M. Lange, Ewelina Makulska-Gertruda, Yukiko Nakamura, Andreas Reissmann, Shigehiko Kanaya, and Joachim Hauser. "Ketogenic Diets and Alzheimer's Disease." *Food Science and Human Wellness* 6, no. 1 (2017): 1–9. https://doi .org/10.1016/j.fshw.2016.10.003.

"Larger, Earlier Drug Trials Needed to Fight Alzheimer's." Technology Networks, July 2019. https://www.technologynetworks.com/neuro science/news/larger-earlier-drug-trials-needed-to-fight-alzheimers -321649.

Laws, Keith R., Karen Irvine, and Tim M. Gale. "Sex Differences in Alzheimer's Disease." *Current Opinion in Psychiatry* 31, no. 2 (2018): 133–139. https://doi.org/10.1097/YCO.0000000000000401.

Leggieri, Melissa, Michael H. Thaut, Luis Fornazzari, Tom A. Schweizer, Joseph Barfett, David G. Munoz, and Corinne E. Fischer. "Music Intervention Approaches for Alzheimer's Disease: A Review of the Literature." *Frontiers in Neuroscience* 13, no. 132 (2019): 1–8. https://doi.org/10.3389/fnins.2019.00132.

The Lewin Group. *Process Evaluation of the Older Americans Act Title III-E National Family Caregiver Support Program: Final Report*, 2016. https://acl.gov/sites/default/files/programs/2017-02/NFCSP _Final_Report-update.pdf.

Liao, Huan, Z. Zhu, and Y. Peng. "Potential Utility of Retinal Imaging for Alzheimer's Disease: A Review." *Frontiers in Aging Neuroscience* 10 (2018): 188. https://doi.org/10.3389/fnagi.2018.00188.

Liew, Tau Ming and Cia Sin Lee. "Reappraising the Efficacy and Acceptability of Multicomponent Interventions for Caregiver Depression in Dementia: The Utility of Network Meta-Analysis." *The Gerontologist* 59, no. 4 (2019): 380–392. https://doi.org/10.1093/geront/gny061.

Liu, Zheng, Qian-lin Chen, and Yu-ying Sun. "Mindfulness Training for Psychological Stress in Family Caregivers of Persons with Dementia: A Systematic Review and Meta-Analysis of Randomized Controlled Trials." *Dove Press Journal: Clinical Interventions in Aging* 12 (2017): 1521–1529. https://doi.org/10.2147/CIA.S146213.

Lök, Neslihan, Kerime Bademli, and Alime Selçuk-Tosun. "The Effect of Reminiscence Therapy on Cognitive Functions, Depression, and Quality of Life in Alzheimer Patients: Randomized Controlled Trial." *International Journal of Geriatric Psychiatry* 34, no. 1 (2019): 47–53. https://doi.org/10.1002/gps.4980.

Lourida, Ilianna, Eilis Hannon, Thomas J. Littlejohns, Kenneth M. Langa, Elina Hyppönen, Elzbieta Kuzma, and David J. Llewellyn. "Association of Lifestyle and Genetic Risk with Incidence of Dementia." *JAMA* 322, no. 5 (2019): 430–437. https://doi.org/10.1001/jama.2019.9879.

Lu, Linda C. and Juergen H. Bludau. *Alzheimer's Disease.* Santa Barbara, CA: Greenwood, 2011.

Ma, Mandy, Diana Dorstyn, Lynn Ward, and Shaun Prentice. "Alzheimer's Disease and Caregiving: A Meta-Analytic Review Comparing the Mental Health of Primary Carers to Controls." *Aging Mental Health* 22, no. 11 (2018): 1395–1405. https://doi.org/10.1080/13607863.2017 .1370689.

Mandrekar-Colucci, Shweta and Gary E. Landreth. "Microglia and Inflammation in Alzheimer's Disease." *CNS & Neurological Disorders Drug Targets* 9, no. 2 (2010): 156–167. https://doi.org/10.2174/187152 710791012071.

Matura, S., J. Fleckenstein, R. Deichmann, T. Engeroff, E. Füzéki, E. Hattingen, R. Hellweg, et al. "Effects of Aerobic Exercise on Brain Metabolism and Grey Matter Volume in Older Adults: Results of the Randomised Controlled SMART Trial." *Translational Psychiatry* 7, no. 7 (2017): e1172. https://doi.org/10.1038/tp.2017.135.

Maurer, Konrad, Stephan Volk, and Hector Gerbaldo. "Auguste D and Alzheimer's Disease." *The Lancet* 349 (1997): 1546–1549. https:// doi.org/10.1016/S0140-6736(96)10203-8.

"Medications for Memory, Cognition and Dementia-Related Behaviors." *Alzheimer's Disease and Dementia.* https://www.alz.org/alzheimers -dementia/treatments/medications-for-memory.

Merz, Beverly. "Can You Recognize the Warning Signs of Alzheimer's Disease?" Harvard Health, May 30, 2017. https://www.health .harvard.edu/mind-and-mood/can-you-recognize-the-warning-signs -of-alzheimers-disease.

Mitolo, Micaela, Caterina Tonon, Chiara La Morgia, Claudia Testa, Valerio Carelli, and Raffaele Lodi. "Effects of Light Treatment on Sleep, Cognition, Mood, and Behavior in Alzheimer's Disease: A Systematic Review." *Dementia and Geriatric Cognitive Disorders* 46, no. 5–6 (2018): 371–384. https://doi.org/10.1159/000494921.

Moulder, Krista L., B. Joy Snider, Susan L. Mills, Virginia D. Buckles, Anna M. Santacruz, Randall J. Bateman, and John C. Morris. "Dominantly Inherited Alzheimer Network: Facilitating Research and Clinical

Trials." *Alzheimer's Research & Therapy* 5, no. 5 (2013): 48. https:// doi.org/10.1186/alzrt213.

Müller, Stephan, Oliver Preische, Hamid R. Sohrabi, Susanne Gräber, Mathias Jucker, John M. Ringman, Ralph N. Martins, et al. "Relationship Between Physical Activity, Cognition, and Alzheimer Pathology in Autosomal Dominant Alzheimer's Disease." *Alzheimer's & Dementia* 14, no. 11 (2018): 1427–1437. https://doi.org /10.1016/j.jalz.2018.06.3059.

Musiek, Erik S., Meghana Bhimasani, Margaret A. Zangrilli, John C. Morris, David M. Holtzman, and Yo-El S. Ju. "Circadian Rest-Activity Pattern Changes in Aging and Preclinical Alzheimer Disease." *JAMA Neurology* 75, no. 5 (2018): 582–590. https://doi.org/10.1001 /jamaneurol.2017.4719.

"Nanodevices for the Brain Could Thwart Formation of Alzheimer's Plaques." Neuroscience News, April 30, 2020. http://www.neuro sciencenews.com/nanodevice-amyloid-beta-16294.

"National Poll on Healthy Aging. Dementia Caregivers: Juggling, Delaying and Looking Forward." University of Michigan's Institute for Healthcare Policy and Innovation. November 2017. http://www .healthyagingpoll.org/sites/default/files/2017-10/NPHA_Caregivers -Report-PROOF_101817_v2.pdf.

Neubauer, Noelannah A., Peyman Azad-Khaneghah, Antonio Miguel-Cruz, and Lili Liu. "What Do We Know about Strategies to Manage Dementia-related Wandering? A Scoping Review." *Alzheimer's & Dementia: Diagnosis, Assessment & Disease Monitoring* 10, no. 1 (2018): 615–628.

Ngolab, Jennifer, Patrick Honma, and Robert A. Rissman. "Reflections on the Utility of the Retina as a Biomarker for Alzheimer's Disease: A Literature Review." *Neurology and Therapy* 8, no. S2 (2019): 57–72. https://doi.org/10.1007/s40120-019-00173-4.

Nitkin, Karen. "Alzheimer's Disease: Frustration and Hope." Johns Hopkins Medicine, November 19, 2018. https://www.hopkinsmedicine .org/news/articles/alzheimers-disease-frustration-and-hope.

Nobis, Lisa and Masud Husain. "Apathy in Alzheimer's Disease." *Current Opinion in Behavioral Sciences* 22 (2018): 7–13. https://doi.org /10.1016/j.cobeha.2017.12.007.

Noordzij, Marlies, Friedo W. Dekker, Carmine Zoccali, and Kitty J. Jager. "Measures of Disease Frequency: Prevalence and Incidence." *Nephron Clinical Practice* 115, no. 1 (2010): c17–c20. https://doi.org /10.1159/000286345.

"Number of People with Dementia Will Double in Twenty Years." Neuroscience News, October 29, 2019. https://neurosciencenews.com /dementia-doubling-15145.

"Our Nation's Workforce Shortage." Eldercare Workforce Alliance. https://eldercareworkforce.org/workforce-shortage.

Oxford, Alexandra E., Erica S. Stewart, and Troy T. Rohn. "Clinical Trials in Alzheimer's Disease: A Hurdle in the Path of Remedy." *International Journal of Alzheimer's Disease* (2020): 1–13. https://doi.org/10.1155/2020/5380346.

Palmqvist, Sebastian, Shorena Janelidze, Erik Stomrud, Henrik Zetterberg, Johann Karl, Katharina Zink, Tobias Bittner, et al. "Performance of Fully Automated Plasma Assays as Screening Tests for Alzheimer Disease–Related β-Amyloid Status." *JAMA Neurology* 76, no. 9 (2019): 1060–1069. https://doi.org/10.1001/jamaneurol.2019.1632.

Pardridge, William M. "Alzheimer's Disease Drug Development and the Problem of the Blood-Brain Barrier." *Alzheimer's & Dementia* 5, no. 5 (2009): 427–432. https://doi.org/10.1016/j.jalz.2009.06.003.

Peck, Katlyn J., Todd A. Girard, Frank A. Russo, and Alexandra J. Fiocco. "Music and Memory in Alzheimer's Disease and the Potential Underlying Mechanisms." *Journal of Alzheimer's Disease* 51, no. 4 (2016): 949–959. https://doi.org/10.3233/jad-150998.

Perlmutter, David. *Grain Brain: The Surprising Truth about Wheat, Carbs, and Sugar—Your Brain's Silent Killers.* New York: Little, Brown Spark, 2015.

Perlmutter, David. "Taking Control of the Alzheimer's Gene." DrPerlmutter.com, April 23, 2018. http://www.drperlmutter.com/taking-control-of-the-alzheimers-gene.

Port, Cynthia L., Sheryl Zimmerman, Christianna S. Williams, Debra Dobbs, John S. Preisser, and Sharon Wallace Williams. "Families Filling the Gap: Comparing Family Involvement for Assisted Living and Nursing Home Residents with Dementia." *Gerontologist* 45, no. 1 (2005): 87–95. https://doi.org/10.1093/geront/45.suppl_1.87.

Porteri, Corinna. "Advance Directives as a Tool to Respect Patients' Values and Preferences: Discussion on the Case of Alzheimer's Disease." *BMC Medical Ethics* 19, no. 1 (2018): 9. https://doi.org/10.1186/s12910-018-0249-6.

Poulin, Michael J., Stephanie L. Brown, Peter A. Ubel, Dylan M. Smith, Aleksandra Jankovic, and Kenneth M. Langa. "Does a Helping Hand Mean a Heavy Heart? Helping Behavior and Well-Being among Spouse Caregivers." *Psychology and Aging* 25, no. 1 (2010): 108–117. https://doi.org/10.1037/a0018064.

Qian, Jing, Frank J. Wolters, Alexa Beiser, Mary Haan, M. Arfan Ikram, Jason Karlawish, Jessica B. Langbaum, et al. "*APOE*-related Risk of Mild Cognitive Impairment and Dementia for Prevention Trials:

An Analysis of Four Cohorts." *PLoS Medicine* 14, no. 3 (2017): e1002254. https://doi.org/10.1371/journal.pmed.1002254.

Rabarison, Kristina M., Erin D. Bouldin, Connie L. Bish, Lisa C. McGuire, Christopher A. Taylor, Kurt J. Greenlund. "The Economic Value of Informal Caregiving for Persons with Dementia: Results from 38 States, the District of Columbia, and Puerto Rico, 2015 and 2016 BRFSS." *American Journal of Public Health* 108, no. 10 (2018): 1370–1377. https://doi.org/10.2105/AJPH.2018.304573.

Rajan, Kumar B., Jennifer Weuve, Lisa L. Barnes, Robert S. Wilson, and Denis A. Evans. "Prevalence and Incidence of Clinically Diagnosed Alzheimer's Disease Dementia from 1994 to 2012 in a Population Study." *Alzheimer's & Dementia* 15, no. 1 (2018): 1–7. https://doi.org/10.1016/j.jalz.2018.07.216.

Reagan, Ronald. "Reagan's Letter Announcing His Alzheimer's Diagnosis." Ronald Reagan Presidential Library & Museum, November 5, 1994. https://www.reaganlibrary.gov/reagans/ronald-reagan/reagans-letter-announcing-his-alzheimers-diagnosis.

"Reducing Early Brain Inflammation Could Slow Alzheimer's Progression." Neuroscience News, April 27, 2020. https://neurosciencenews.com/alzheimers-brain-inflammation-16251.

Reiman, Eric M., Jessica B. S. Langbaum, Adam S. Fleisher, Richard J. Caselli, Kewei Chen, Napatkamon Ayutyanont, Yakeel T. Quiroz, et al. "Alzheimer's Prevention Initiative: A Plan to Accelerate the Evaluation of Presymptomatic Treatments." *Journal of Alzheimer's Disease* 26 Suppl 3, no. s3 (2011): 321–329. https://doi.org/10.3233/JAD-2011-0059.

Riffin, Catherine, Peter H. Van Ness, Jennifer L. Wolff, and Terri Fried. "Family and Other Unpaid Caregivers and Older Adults with and without Dementia and Disability." *Journal of the American Geriatrics Society* 65, no. 8 (2017): 1821–1828. https://doi.org/10.1111/jgs.14910.

Robson, David. "How Flashing Lights Could Treat Alzheimer's Disease." BBC Future, May 19, 2020. https://www.bbc.com/future/article/20200519-alzheimers-can-flashing-lights-provide-a-new-treatment.

Rotolto, Candace. "Medical Tests Used to Diagnose Alzheimer's Disease." *Aging Care.* https://www.agingcare.com/articles/alzheimers-dementia-testing-149186.htm.

Russell-Williams, Jesse, Wafa Jaroudi, Tania Perich, Siobhan Hoscheidt, Mohamad El Haj, and Ahmed A. Moustafa. "Mindfulness and Meditation: Treating Cognitive Impairment and Reducing Stress in Dementia." *Reviews in the Neurosciences* 2, no. 1 (2018): 791–804. https://doi.org/10.1515/revneuro-2017-0066.

Sapkota, Shraddha, Tao Huan, Tran Tran, Jiamin Zheng, Richard Camicioli, Liang Li, and Roger A. Dixon. "Alzheimer's Biomarkers from Multiple Modalities Selectively Discriminate Clinical Status: Relative Importance of Salivary Metabolomics Panels, Genetic, Lifestyle, Cognitive, Functional Health and Demographic Risk Markers." *Frontiers in Aging Neuroscience* 2, no. 10 (2018): 296. https://doi.org/10.3389/fnagi.2018.00296.

Saunders, A. M., W. J. Strittmatter, D. Schmechel, P. H. St. George-Hyslop, M. A. Pericak-Vance, S. H. Joo, B. L. Rosi, et al. "Association of Apolipoprotein E Allele Epsilon 4 with Late-onset Familial and Sporadic Alzheimer's Disease." *Neurology* 43, no. 8 (1993): 1467–1472. https://doi.org/10.1212/WNL.43.8.1467.

Schilling, Melissa A. "Unraveling Alzheimer's: Making Sense of the Relationship between Diabetes and Alzheimer's Disease." *Journal of Alzheimer's Disease: JAD* 51, no. 4 (2016): 961–977. https://doi.org/10.3233/JAD-150980.

Schindler, Suzanne E., James G. Bollinger, Vitaliy Ovod, Kwasi G. Mawuenyega, Yan Li, Brian A. Gordon, David M. Holtzman, et al. "High Precision Plasma Amyloid-β 42/40 Predicts Current and Future Brain Amyloidosis." *Neurology* 93, no. 17 (2019): 1647–1659. https://doi.org/10.1212/WNL.0000000000008081.

Schulz, Richard, Steven H. Belle, Sara J. Czaja, Kathleen A. McGinnis, Alan Stevens, Song Zhang. "Long-Term Care Placement of Dementia Patients and Caregiver Health and Well-Being." *JAMA* 292, no. 8 (2004): 961–967. https://doi.org/10.1001/jama.292.8.961; https://jamanetwork.com/journals/jama/fullarticle/199315.

Schulz, Richard, Aaron B. Mendelsohn, William E. Haley, Diane Mahoney, Rebecca S. Allen, Song Zhang, Larry Thompson, et al. "End-of-Life Care and the Effects of Bereavement on Family Caregivers of Persons with Dementia." *New England Journal of Medicine* 349, no. 20 (2003): 1936–1942. https://doi.org/10.1056/NEJMsa035373.

Sharma, Nikhil, Joseph Classen, and Leonardo G. Cohen. "Neural Plasticity and Its Contribution to Functional Recovery." *Neurological Rehabilitation* 110 (2013): 3–12. https://doi.org/10.1016/b978-0-444-52901-5.00001-0.

"Sleep Loss Linked to Increase in Alzheimer's Plaques." *ScienceDaily.* September 25, 2009. http://www.sciencedaily.com/releases/2009/09/090924141742.htm.

Sommerlad, Andrew, Séverine Sabia, Archana Singh-Manoux, Glyn Lewis, and Gill Livingston. "Association of Social Contact with Dementia and Cognition: 28-Year Follow-Up of the Whitehall II Cohort Study." *PLOS Medicine* 1, no. 8 (2019): e1002862. https://doi.org/10.1371/journal.pmed.1002862.

Spillman, Brenda C., Jennifer Wolff, Vicki A. Freedman, and Judith D. Kasper. "Informal Caregiving for Older Americans: An Analysis of the 2011 National Health and Aging Trends Study." U.S. Department of Health and Human Services, April 1, 2014. https://aspe .hhs.gov/report/informal-caregiving-older-americans-analysis-2011 -national-study-caregiving.

Stall, Nathan M., Sanghun J. Kim, Kate A. Hardacre, Prakesh S. Shah, Sharon E. Straus, Susan E. Bronskill, Lisa M. Lix, et al. "Association of Informal Caregiver Distress with Health Outcomes of Community-Dwelling Dementia Care Recipients: A Systematic Review." *Journal of the American Geriatrics Society* 67, no. 3 (2019): 609–617. https:// doi.org/10.1111/jgs.15690.

Stern, Yaakov. "Cognitive Reserve in Ageing and Alzheimer's Disease." *Lancet Neurology* 11, no. 11 (2012): 1006–1012. https://doi.org /10.1016/S1474-4422(12)70191-6.

Stone, Robyn I. "Factors Affecting the Future of Family Caregiving in the United States." In *Family Caregiving in the New Normal*, edited by Joseph E. Gaugler and Robert L. Kane, 57–77. San Diego, CA: Elsevier, 2015. https://doi.org/10.1016/B978-0-12-417046-9.00006-4.

"Stress Can Impair Memory, Reduce Brain Size in Middle Age." *ScienceDaily*, October 25, 2018. https://www.sciencedaily.com/releases /2018/10/181025084043.htm.

Strobel, Gabrielle. "Early Onset Familial AD." Alzforum. September 9, 2020. https://www.alzforum.org/early-onset-familial-ad/overview /what-early-onset-familial-alzheimer-disease-efad.

Supe, Ujjwala and Jayant Supe. "Alzheimer: A Disease of Brain." *International Journal of Engineering and Creative Science* 1, no. 1 (2018). http://ijecs.net/Archive/IJECS-2.pdf.

Tarasoff-Conway, Jenna M., Roxana O. Carare, Ricardo S. Osorio, Lidia Glodzik, Tracy Butler, Els Fieremans, Leon Axel, et al. "Clearance Systems in the Brain: Implications for Alzheimer disease." *Nature Reviews. Neurology* 11, no. 8 (2015): 457–470. https://doi.org/10 .1038/nrneurol.2015.119.

Toepper, Max. "Dissociating Normal Aging from Alzheimer's Disease: A View from Cognitive Neuroscience." *Journal of Alzheimer's Disease* 57, no. 2 (2017): 331–352. https://doi.org/10.3233/JAD-161099.

Trafton, Anne. "Brain Wave Stimulation May Improve Alzheimer's Symptoms." MIT News, March 14, 2019. https://news.mit.edu/2019 /brain-wave-stimulation-improve-alzheimers-0314.

"Treatments and Research." Alzheimer's Association. https://www.alz.org /alzheimers-dementia/research_progress/treatment-horizon.

Triplett, Patrick, Betty S. Black, Hilary Phillips, Sarah Richardson Fahrendorf, Jack Schwartz, Andrew F. Angelino, Danielle Anderson, et al.

"Content of Advance Directives for Individuals with Advanced Dementia." *Journal of Aging and Health* 20, no. 5 (2008): 583–596. https://doi.org/10.1177/0898264308317822.

"2021 Alzheimer's Disease Facts and Figures." *Alzheimer's & Dementia* 17, no. 3 (2020): 327–426. https://doi.org/10.1002/alz.12328.

"Understanding Genetics and Alzheimer's Disease." Alzheimer Society, August 2014. https://archive.alzheimer.ca/sites/default/files/files /national/research/understanding_genetics_e.pdf.

"The United States Will Soon Be Bigger, Older, and More Diverse." APM Research Lab. https://www.apmresearchlab.org/blog/the-united -states-will-soon-be-bigger-older-and-more-diverse.

Van Cauwenberghe, Caroline, Christine Van Broeckhoven, and Kristel Sleegers. "The Genetic Landscape of Alzheimer Disease: Clinical Implications and Perspectives." *Genetics in Medicine* 18, no. 5 (2016): 421–430. https://doi.org/10.1038/gim.2015.117.

Vaz, Miguel, and Samuel Silvestre. "Alzheimer's Disease: Recent Treatment Strategies." *European Journal of Pharmacology* 887 (2020): 173554. https://doi.org/10.1016/j.ejphar.2020.173554.

Verreault, René, Danielle Laurin, Joan Lindsay, and Gaston De Serres. "Past Exposure to Vaccines and Subsequent Risk of Alzheimer's Disease." *CMAJ: Canadian Medical Association Journal* 165, no. 11 (2001): 1495–1498.

Voordouw, A. C. G., M. C. J. M. Sturkenboom, J. P. Dieleman, Th. Stijnen, D. J. Smith, J. van der Lei, and Bruno H. Ch. Stricker. "Annual Revaccination Against Influenza and Mortality Risk in Community-Dwelling Elderly Persons." *JAMA* 292, no. 17 (2004): 2089–2095. https://doi.org/10.1001/jama.292.17.2089.

Warshaw, Gregg A. and Elizabeth J. Bragg. "Preparing the Health Care Workforce to Care for Adults with Alzheimer's Disease and Related Dementias." *Health Affairs* 33, no. 4 (2014): 633–641. https://doi .org/10.1377/hlthaff.2013.1232.

Washington University School of Medicine. "Blood Test Is Highly Accurate at Identifying Alzheimer's before Symptoms Arise." *ScienceDaily*. https://www.sciencedaily.com/releases/2019/08/190801162144 .htm.

Weir, K. "Keeping Dementia at Bay." *Monitor on Psychology*, 48, no. 7 (2017). http://www.apa.org/monitor/2017/07-08/cover-dementia.

Wells, Rebecca Erwin, Gloria Y. Yeh, Catherine E. Kerr, Jennifer Wolkin, Roger B. Davis, Ying Tan, Rosa Spaeth, et al. "Meditation's Impact on Default Mode Network and Hippocampus in Mild Cognitive Impairment: A Pilot Study." *Neuroscience Letters* 556 (2013): 15–19. https://doi.org/10.1016/j.neulet.2013.10.001.

Winslow, Ron. "The Future of Alzheimer's Treatment May Be Enlisting the Immune System." *Medium*, June 4, 2019. https://onezero.medium.com/the-future-of-alzheimers-treatment-may-be-enlisting-the-immune-system-d4de95ac1cff.

Włodarek, Dariusz. "Role of Ketogenic Diets in Neurodegenerative Diseases (Alzheimer's Disease and Parkinson's Disease)." *Nutrients* 11, no. 1 (2019): 169. https://doi.org/10.3390/nu11010169.

Wolff, Jennifer L., John Mulcahy, Jin Huang, David L. Roth, Kenneth Covinsky, and Judith D. Kasper. "Family Caregivers of Older Adults, 1999–2015: Trends in Characteristics, Circumstances, and Role-Related Appraisal." *The Gerontologist* 58, no. 6 (2018): 1021–1032. https://doi.org/10.1093/geront/gnx093.

Yang, Hyun Duk, Do Han Kim, Sang Bong Lee, and Linn Derg Young. "History of Alzheimer's Disease." *Dementia and Neurocognitive Disorders* 15, no. 4 (2016): 115–121. https://doi.org/10.12779/dnd.2016.15.4.115.

Yazar, Tamer, Hülya Olgun Yazar, Esra Yancar Demir, Fatih Özdemir, Soner Çankaya, and Özgür Enginyurt. "Assessment of the Mental Health of Carers According to the Stage of Patients with Diagnosis of Alzheimer-Type Dementia." *Neurological Sciences* 39 (2018): 903–908. https://doi.org/10.1007/s10072-018-3293-6.

Yiannopoulou, Konstantina G. and Sokratis G. Papageorgiou. "Current and Future Treatments in Alzheimer Disease: An Update." *Journal of Central Nervous System Disease* 12 (2020). https://doi.org/10.1177/1179573520907397.

Yu, Rongqin, Anya Topiwala, Robin Jacoby, and Seena Fazel. "Aggressive Behaviors in Alzheimer Disease and Mild Cognitive Impairment: Systematic Review and Meta-Analysis." *American Journal of Geriatric Psychiatry* 27, no. 3 (2019): 290–300. https://doi.org/10.1016/j.jagp.2018.10.008.

Index

Abuse, 85
Acetylcholine, 27, 51, 129
Acetylcholinesterase, 52, 122
Activities of daily living (ADLs), 41, 68, 79, 81, 108
ADDvac-1 vaccine, 127
Aducanumab (Aduhelm), 20, 127
Advanced age, 28, 103
African American, 7, 32, 78
Age-related macular degeneration, 41
Aggression, 13, 22, 35, 53–54, 69, 75, 81
Agitation, 40, 53, 58, 69, 75, 81–82, 109, 140, 143
Alcohol, 3, 40
Allele, 29–30, 93, 95
Alternative treatments, 54, 143
Alzheimer, Alois, 11, 15, 20, 48
Alzheimer's Association, 7; behavioral disturbances, 73, 75; caregiving, 77–78, 80, 82, 85–86, 88; diagnosis, 50; dietary factors, 96; memory problems, 37; milestones, 16–17, 19; myths, 8; plaques and tangles, 24; treatments, 125; what to do, 42
Alzheimer's dementia, 2–3, 117, 118, 127
Amyloid beta, 25; blood tests, 120; diagnostic methods, 119–120; sensory therapies, 58; sleep, 100–101; treatments, 126–128

Amyloid hypothesis, 26, 121, 126
Amyloid plaques, 2; causes, 26; dietary factors, 95; disease discovery, 14; identifying, 48; onset, 22; risk factors, 29–30, 33; sex differences, 6; treatments, 129, 132; typical aging, 65
Amyloid precursor protein (APP), 18–19, 22, 24–26, 123, 126
Animal studies, 101, 128
Antagonist drugs, 128–129
Anthocyanidins, 96
Antibodies, 126–128
Antipsychotic drug, 53–54
Anxiety, 40, 53, 58–60, 64, 69, 81–82, 85–86
Aphasia, 76
Apolipoprotein (APOE) ε4 gene, 6–7, 18, 23, 25–26, 28–30, 49, 93, 95, 98–99, 102, 120, 127, 129
Appetite, 40, 53, 73, 84–85
Aricept, 27, 52
Asian, 78
Assessment, 4, 45, 47–48, 67, 88, 105, 115, 120, 125, 133, 136–137, 141; battery, 48, 52, 56, 136; biomarker, 4, 67, 120; cognitive, 55, 98, 118, 122; neuroimaging, 48–49, 119; neurological, 47–48, 118; neuropsychological, 50; noninvasive, 3, 49, 125, 130; physical, 118; self, 105

Assistance, 14, 38, 47, 55, 69, 71, 77, 79–82, 84, 86–87, 142
Assisted living, 70, 71, 75, 79, 81, 145
Atrophy, 6, 26, 28, 50, 61, 102–103, 132
Attention, 7, 14, 37, 46–47, 50–51, 54, 58–60, 67, 93, 103, 129–131, 136
Autobiographical memory, 56, 58, 66
Autoimmune response, 94, 126
Autonomic nervous system, 58
Autonomy, 59, 75, 110–111
Autopsy, 3, 14, 29, 33, 59, 75, 95, 110–111, 124
Autosomal-dominant Alzheimer's disease, 22
Awareness (cognitive), 39, 59, 68, 70, 103, 139; awareness (of the disease), 15–19
Axon, 25–26
Axona, 97

Bathing, 38, 41, 68–69, 79, 81, 108, 146
Beta secretase, 25
Biomarker, 4, 20, 36, 48–49, 67, 100–101, 117–122, 125, 130
Blood-brain barrier, 96, 123, 129, 132, 133
Blood test, 120–121
Bloodstream, 29, 70, 93–94, 96, 100, 121, 133
Blue-light autofluorescence (BAF), 123
Bowel control, 36, 70, 143
Brain imaging, 19, 22, 45, 49, 98, 119–120, 123–125, 136
Brain-derived neurotropic factor (BDNF), 65, 98–99
Burden of disease, 4, 75, 82–83, 87–88, 131, 145–146

C9ORF72, 27
Cancer, 18, 49, 91, 129
Capillary, 102, 129, 133
Carbohydrates, 83, 93–95, 97, 137
Cardiovascular disease, 29–30
Caregiving, 53, 55, 68–69, 73–90, 110, 112, 139–141, 143–146

Caretaker, 68, 71, 73, 75, 87–88, 112–113, 130
Cataracts, 41
Cell, 23–26, 28, 97, 123, 125, 127
Centers for Disease Control and Prevention (CDC), 1, 19, 32
Central nervous system, 123, 129
Cerebral cortex, 12, 14
Cerebrospinal fluid (CSF), 22, 36, 100–101, 117, 122, 130
Cerebrovascular, 3, 17, 117, 124
Cholesterol, 29–30, 93, 96
Cholinergic, 27
Cholinesterase inhibitor, 27, 51, 52, 56
Chromosome, 18, 22–23, 29, 93
Chronic traumatic encephalopathy (CTE), 3, 33
Chronic stress, 82, 103–104
Cingulate cortex, 130
Circadian rhythms, 101
Clinical interview, 47–48
Clinical trial, 17–19, 52, 55, 119–120, 125–127, 129–133
Cognex, 18
Cognition, 37, 47, 50, 53–59, 70, 75, 97–98, 108, 118, 122, 129–131
Cognitive decline, 6; awareness, 15–16, 20; behavioral disturbances, 73, 75; complications, 72; conditions, 30–31; diagnosis, 46–47, 50; exercise, 98; interventions, 55–56; mental engagement, 101; prevention, 92–96; prognosis, 72; stress, 104; treatments, 51, 60, 126–127, 129, 132; typical aging, 63–66
Cognitive rehabilitation, 54–55
Cognitive reserve, 32, 93, 102, 117
Cognitive stimulation, 54–56
Cognitive training, 54–55
Communication, 2, 6, 26, 41, 52, 56–57, 75, 78, 81, 100, 109, 130
Community, 7, 12, 14, 72, 79, 83–84, 145
Comorbid, 7, 50
Computerized tomography (CT), 49, 119, 136

Concentration, 69, 85
Confusion, 3, 46–47, 53, 57, 69, 78, 139
Consciousness, 2–3
Consultation, 40, 135–136
Controversies, 107, 109, 111, 113
Coordination, 47–48, 72, 88
Coping, 12, 84, 86–87, 89, 128, 146
Cortical thickness, 103
Costs, 71, 75, 80, 87–88, 109, 119, 121, 125, 127
Counseling, 56–57, 88, 145
Cystic fibrosis, 24, 92

Daily living skills, 2, 52, 68, 70, 109
DASH diet, 83, 96
Death, 1–2, 8, 14, 19, 30, 36, 73–74, 76, 85, 92, 94, 97, 139
Decision-making, 38, 45–46, 81, 108–111, 131, 142
Degeneration, 11–12, 17, 41, 50–51, 98, 121, 123
Delirium, 40–41
Delusions, 14, 36, 53–54, 69, 112
Dendrites, 25, 27
Deoxyribonucleic acid (DNA), 23, 28
Depression, 3, 40, 42, 49–50, 53–54, 56–60, 64, 72–75, 81–83, 85, 89, 111, 128, 140–141
Deter, Auguste, 12–14, 16, 19
Diabetes, 1, 7, 30, 42, 71, 94–95, 98, 117, 144
Diagnostic and Statistical Manual of Mental Disorders (DSM-5), 46–47
Diagnostic criteria, 3, 46–47
Diet, 31, 76, 83, 93–98, 105, 125, 137, 143
Differential diagnosis, 49–50
Disorientation, 14, 38, 47, 57, 64, 138, 143
Distraction, 37, 75, 131
Donepezil, 27, 52–53, 76
Double-blind study, 52, 60
Dressing, 8, 35, 38, 40–41, 79, 81, 87, 135, 140
Driving, 35, 38, 41, 139, 143
Drowsiness, 53

Dysfunction, 28, 33, 37, 64, 68, 126
Dysphoria, 73

Early-onset Alzheimer's, 8, 21–24, 27, 29, 53, 57, 92, 99, 126
Early-onset familial Alzheimer's disease (EOFAD), 21, 23–24, 92
Early stage of Alzheimer's, 27, 35, 28, 53, 55, 60, 66–67, 89, 119, 123, 132, 136–137, 139, 143
Education, 6, 32, 78–79, 88, 117
Effectiveness, 19, 53–54, 57–58, 133
Efficacy, 98, 115, 125, 126, 128, 129, 131, 133
Electromagnetic, 130
Emotions, 2, 47, 57, 74, 80, 83
Empathy, 51, 75
Encephalopathy, 3, 33
Energy, 6, 21, 28, 30, 94, 96–97, 100, 133, 140
Engagement, 30–32, 72, 75, 99–103, 105, 135
Entorhinal cortex, 26
Enzyme, 52, 95, 126
Enzyme-linked immunosorbent assay (ELISA), 121–122
Epilepsy, 12
Episodic memory, 6, 50, 59, 65–66
Ethnic, 7, 32, 78–79
Etiology, 48, 50, 118
Evaluation, 45, 53, 136–137, 139
Executive function, 32, 47, 54, 69
Exelon, 52
Exercise, 30–31, 75, 83–84, 86, 91, 93, 98–100, 105, 137
Expenditures, 71, 87–88

Falling, 32, 41, 69, 74, 76, 85
Familial Alzheimer's disease (FAD), 24
Farsightedness, 125
Fatigue, 40, 49, 52, 136, 144, 145
Feeding, 47, 68, 70, 76, 81, 110
Feelings, 25, 40, 57, 59, 72–73, 83, 89, 102, 109, 138, 140, 144–145
Finances, 37, 68, 81, 87, 145
Flavonoids, 96

Flu, 8; influenza, 1, 8
fMRI. *See* Functional magnetic
    resonance imagery (fMRI)
Food and Drug Administration (FDA),
    9, 18, 20, 51, 53, 125–128, 130
Forgetting, 8, 35–39, 63, 65, 67–68, 70,
    76, 83–84, 135, 138–139, 141
Fornix, 131–132
Frontal lobe, 50, 70, 131, 133, 152, 153
Frontotemporal degradation, 50, 51,
    121
Frontotemporal dementia, 28, 50–51,
    121
Fruits, 31, 83, 96
Frustration, 40, 49, 65, 75, 85, 109, 135,
    138–141, 145
Functional brain imaging, 49
Functional decline, 57, 69, 131
Functional magnetic resonance
    imagery (fMRI), 49, 61

Gait, 70, 76, 136
Galantamine, 52
Gamma secretase, 25, 126
Gamma wave, 132
Gene(s), 6–7, 18–19, 21–30, 49, 92–93,
    95, 99, 102, 120, 127
Genetic mutation, 22, 24, 26–27, 92, 99
Genetics, 6–7, 19–24, 27–28, 32,
    48–50, 71, 91–93, 95, 98–100, 104,
    109, 125, 137
Genetic variant, 6–7, 28, 49, 92, 93, 95,
    98–99
Genome, 23, 92
Genome-wide association study
    (GWAS), 23
Genotype, 6, 48–49, 92
Geras, 15
Geriatric, 54, 75, 80, 85, 87–88,
    110–111
Gerontology, 80
Glaucoma, 41
Glucose, 30, 94, 96–97
Glutamate, 52
Glycogen, 96–97
Glymphatic system, 100

Grains, 31, 83, 96–97
Gray matter, 67, 103
Grief, 12, 89, 112, 146
Grooming, 81
Guilt, 64, 84, 144, 146

Habits: eating, 96; lifestyle, 31; sleep,
    137; social, 56
Hallucinations, 14, 36, 50, 53–54, 69
Hearing, 40, 47, 54, 69, 142
Hemorrhage, 119, 124
Herbs, 96
Heredity, 22–23
Hippocampus, 26, 52, 61, 65, 96, 103
Hippocrates, 15
Hispanic Americans, 7, 32, 78
HIV, 1, 129
Home health aides, 79
Hormones, 6, 82, 94, 103–104
Hospice, 71, 142–143
Huntington's disease, 92
Hydrocephalus, 51
Hygiene, 38, 68, 70, 72–73, 135,
    139–140
Hyperglycemia, 94
Hyperphosphorylation, 6, 127
Hypertension, 30, 60, 144

Immune system, 2, 82, 96, 126–128
Immunodeficiency, 129
Incidence, 4–6
Income, 12, 78, 80, 87
Incontinence, 76, 142
Independence, 3, 17, 35, 37, 47, 55,
    67–69, 72, 74, 109, 129, 131, 137, 143
Infection, 15, 36, 40, 70–71, 76, 94,
    128, 136
Inflammation, 21, 28, 60, 97–98, 100,
    126, 128
Influenza, 1, 8; flu, 8
Informal caretaker, 80, 87, 88, 144
Inherited, 18–19, 21, 22, 24, 92, 127
Injuries, 3, 16, 32, 69–70, 74, 127–128
Insomnia, 52
Instrumental activities of daily living
    (IADL), 81

Insulin resistance, 94–95, 98
Insurance, 47, 119
International Classification of Diseases (ICD), 46–47

Job loss, 64, 78, 146
Judgment, 2, 51, 57, 61, 110, 131, 139

Ketogenic diet, 96–98
Ketosis, 96–97
Kidney disease, 1, 94, 136
Knight Alzheimer's Disease Research Center, 101
Kraepelin, Emil, 14–16

Language: comprehension, 69, 76; loss of, 41, 65
Late-onset Alzheimer's disease, 8, 21–23, 27, 57, 93
Late stage Alzheimer's, 27–28, 50, 53, 58, 63, 70–71, 76, 110, 112, 143
Law, 20, 77–78, 86
Leukemia, 128
Lewy body dementia, 3, 50
Lifestyle changes, 31, 59, 71, 104
Light therapy, 58
Lipid, 133
Loneliness, 72
Longitudinal research, 4–5, 60, 89, 95, 124

Macular degeneration, 41, 124
Magnetic resonance imaging (MRI), 49, 98, 119, 136
Major depressive disorder, 49–50, 64
Major neurocognitive decline, 48
Major neurocognitive disorder, 46
Medicaid, 47, 79, 87
Medicare, 47, 79, 87
Medication, 2, 20, 40, 42, 52–53, 64, 71–76, 78, 80, 87, 108–109, 115, 127, 143–144
Medicine, 11–12, 16, 23, 101, 104, 110, 120
Meditation, 60–61, 86, 103–104
Mediterranean diet, 83, 96

Medium-chain triglycerides (MCTs), 97
Memantine, 52–53, 76, 125
Memories, 26, 37, 56, 58, 66, 83–84, 112, 130, 143
Memory aids, 37
Memory lapses, 67, 135
Memory loss, 2, 8, 11, 18, 22, 26, 29, 31–32, 37, 42, 50, 64, 72, 78, 83, 131
Men, 5–6
Mental health, 47, 82–84, 88, 97
Mental illness, 12, 16
Mental status exam, 45, 48
Metabolite, 122
Microbubble, 132–133
Microglia, 28, 126, 128, 132
Microscope, 12, 17
Microtubule, 25–26, 127
Middle age, 4, 14–15, 30
Middle stage Alzheimer's, 17, 35, 66, 76, 110, 132, 139, 141
Mild cognitive impairment, 3–5, 36, 46, 53, 61, 75, 95, 97, 99, 118–119, 121–124, 127
Mild neurocognitive decline, 46
Mindfulness, 59–60, 84, 89, 103–104
Mindfulness-based stress reduction (MBSR), 60
Mini-Mental State Exam (MMSE), 48, 57–58, 136
Minor neurocognitive disorder, 47–48
Misattributions, 64
Misconceptions, 63–64
Misdiagnosis, 117
Mitochondria, 28, 97
Mobility, 76, 82, 140
Moderate stage Alzheimer's, 17, 52–53, 55, 66, 68–69, 97, 130, 141
Molecules, 21, 26, 28, 100, 127, 129, 132
Money, 12, 32, 35, 38, 40, 55, 69, 72
Montreal Cognitive Assessment (MoCA), 98
Mood, 39–40, 51, 53, 57–58, 61, 64, 68, 72–73, 78, 81, 83, 138–141
Motivation, 2, 45, 73–74, 80

Motor abilities, 45, 47–48, 50, 68, 69–70, 136, 139
Mouth, 70, 142
Movement, 25, 36–37, 47, 49–50, 54, 59, 69–70, 72–73, 99, 136, 143
Multitasking, 66
Music, 56, 58–59, 84, 139
Music therapy, 58–59
Mutation, 18, 22, 24, 26–28, 92, 99
Myths, 8, 63

Namenda, 52, 125
Namzaric, 53
Nanodevices, 133
Nausea, 52, 109
Neighborhood, 38, 99
Neurodegeneration, 14, 104, 120, 123, 127, 129
Neurofibrillary tangles, 2, 6, 15, 17, 24, 48, 65, 72, 100, 126–127, 129
Neurogenesis, 99
Neuroimaging, 20, 48–49, 67, 103; assessment, 48–49, 119
Neuroinflammation, 128
Neurological assessment, 47–48, 118
Neurological disorder, 1, 5, 46–49, 64, 73–74
Neurologist, 136
Neurology, 17, 96, 99, 131
Neuron, 50–52, 99–101, 104, 126–127, 129–130, 132
Neuropathology, 48, 50, 59, 61, 101, 103, 119–124, 127, 130
Neuropathy, 108, 122, 132
Neuroplasticity, 54, 102, 104
Neuroprotein, 99
Neuropsychological assessment, 50
Neuropsychologist, 136
Neuroscience, 59, 121
Neurotoxins, 100
Neurotransmitter, 51–52, 122–123, 129
Nondrug treatments, 107–110
Noninvasive assessment, 3, 49, 125, 130
Nonpharmacological treatment, 51, 53–54, 71, 74, 108–110, 141
Nonverbal memory, 50

Normal aging, 5, 61, 64–66, 139
Nucleus basalis, 51
Nutrients, 2, 25–26, 100

Obesity, 71, 91, 117
Oldest old, 5, 116
Oligomer, 129
Optic nerve, 41, 123–124
Optical coherence tomography (OCT), 123
Orbitofrontal region, 103

Parkinson's disease, 3, 64, 131
Pathogenesis, 58, 61
Pathophysiology, 2–3, 49, 72–73, 127
Peptide, 128, 133
Perceptual-motor ability, 47
Personality changes, 36, 39, 40, 50–51, 68, 78, 81, 86, 139
Pharmacological therapy, 27, 51, 53, 56, 109, 129–130, 132–133, 141
Phosphorylated, 127–128
Physical activity, 30–31, 40, 84, 86, 99, 137
Physical examination, 45, 47, 135
Placebo, 52–54, 97
Planning, 48, 54, 61, 68, 69, 131, 144
Plasma, 100, 120–121
Plasticity (neuroplasticity), 54, 101–102, 104
Pneumonia, 14, 36, 40, 71, 76
Positron emission tomography (PET) scan, 49, 101, 119, 120–121
Preclinical Alzheimer's, 22, 35, 46, 60, 66–67, 101, 118–120, 124–127, 133
Presbyopia, 125
Presenile dementia, 13, 16, 22
Presenilin, 18, 22
Prevalence, 4, 17, 32, 74, 76, 113, 115–118
Processing speed, 37, 50, 66, 122
Prodromal dementia, 46
Prognosis, 63, 65, 67, 69, 71, 73–75, 78
Psychosocial treatment, 54, 56, 57, 107, 109
Psychotherapy, 74
Psychotropic drug, 51

Pythagoras, 15

Race, 7, 32
Radioactive, 119
Randomized controlled trial, 52, 60, 97
Razadyne, 52
Reading, 69, 76, 98, 123, 140
Receptors, 28, 52, 126, 128–129
Redirection, 75, 112
Rehabilitation, 54–56, 71, 74
Relaxation, 58, 86
Religion, 56, 60
Reminiscence therapy, 56–57
Residential care, 72, 84, 86, 88–89
Retina, 41, 120, 123–124
Retinal ganglion cell, 123–124
Retinal imaging, 124–125
Retirement, 31, 146
Rivastigmine, 52

Safety, 55, 74, 125, 128, 133, 137
Saliva tests, 121–122, 125
Sargramostim, 128
Saturated fat, 31, 96
Scanning laser ophthalmoscopy (SLO), 123
Screening test, 48, 58, 98, 121–122, 125, 136
Seizures, 36
Self-esteem, 56, 109
Self-harm, 82
Semantic memory, 6, 65
Semistructured interview, 48
Senile (amyloid) plaques, 2, 6, 14, 18, 19, 22, 24–26, 29–30, 33, 48, 65, 95, 100, 126–127, 132–133
Senilty, 15, 63, 64
Sensory impairment, 48, 136
Sensory therapies, 54, 58–59, 109
Sequential sevens test, 136
Serotonin, 126, 128–129
Severe impairment battery, 52
Severe stage Alzheimer's, 17, 36, 52–54, 66, 70, 112, 141
Showering, 60, 116, 140
Shrinkage (brain), 14, 21, 49, 98, 132, 136

Sickle cell anemia, 24, 92
Side effects, 52–53, 64, 71, 74–75, 109, 130
Single-photon emission computed tomography (SPECT), 119
Sleep, 3, 40, 58, 64, 73, 75, 81, 83, 93, 100–101, 105, 137, 145–146; sleep apnea, 3; sleeplessness, 84–85
Smell, 37, 58–59
Social skills, 55–56
Socioeconomic factors, 7, 32
Spatial skills, 35, 41, 56, 69
Spectrometry, 120, 122
Speech, 36, 48, 57, 76, 136, 142
Spinal tap, 120
Stigma, 19, 46, 81
Stress, 6, 31, 42, 59–61, 64, 75, 78, 82–86, 89, 93, 102–105, 109, 113, 142, 144–145
Stroke, 1, 3, 45, 50, 119
Substance use, 40
Sundowning, 69
Swallowing, 36, 52, 70, 76, 143
Synapse, 25, 27, 54, 104

Tau, 6, 17, 25–28, 33, 67, 100–101, 104, 117, 121–122, 126–130, 132
Temperament, 40
Temporal lobe, 56
Therapy, 6–59, 74, 76, 99, 109–110, 127
Thinking, 2–3, 14, 40, 47, 50–51, 54, 69, 72, 93, 98–99, 110, 135–136
Thyroid, 3
TOMM40 gene, 28
Toxic, 22, 100, 126, 129
Transcranial electromagnetic treatment (TEMT), 130
Traumatic brain injury (TBI), 32–33
Triglycerides, 97
Tumor, 45, 51, 119, 136

Ultrasound, 132–133
Urinary tract infection, 40, 70

Vaccine, 8, 127
Validation therapy, 57

Vascular cognitive impairment, 50
Vascular dementia, 12, 17, 50
Verbal fluency, 54–55
Vision, 41, 47, 54, 70, 85
Visualization, 86

Walking, 11, 39, 59, 69–70, 74, 76, 138, 140, 142–143, 146
Wandering, 36, 53, 69, 74–75, 81–82, 85, 146

Weight loss, 36, 70, 76, 109
Withdrawal, 39–40, 85
Women, 5–6; caregivers, 77; dietary factors, 96
Work, 35; caregivers, 79–80, 83; signs and symptoms, 38–40; stress, 103–104
Workout, 84, 99
World Health Organization (WHO), 46
Writing, 13, 16, 69, 78, 82

About the Authors

Matthew Domico, PsyD, is an assistant professor at Lewis University, Romeoville, Illinois, where he teaches a variety of graduate and undergraduate courses related to clinical psychology. He has experience in providing psychotherapy and assessment services to adults, teens, and children and has worked in hospital, college counseling, and community mental-healthcare settings. His research interests include topics pertaining to health psychology, neurofeedback, student learning, and pedagogy.

Valerie Hill, PhD, is a professor and the undergraduate program director in the Department of Psychology at Lewis University, Romeoville, Illinois, where she teaches a variety of development courses, including one that focuses on Alzheimer's disease. Her scholarly interests include social cognition—in particular, individuals' understanding of social relationships—as well as college student learning and best teaching practices.

Printed in the USA
CPSIA information can be obtained
at www.ICGtesting.com
LVHW010217250823
756247LV00004B/34